WEIGHT LOSS Cookbook

Quick and Easy Recipes for Sustainable Weight Loss

TABLE OF CONTENT

INTRODUCTION
WEIGHT LOSS

The term weight reduction refers to an intentional or unwanted discount in body weight. Losing weight is a proper effect throughout a weight-reduction plan. In comparison, accidental robust and surprising weight loss is a caution signal and might indicate illnesses or parasites. Most human beings in western international locations are mainly involved with their own body weight whilst they are obese and want to reduce excess pounds on the stomach and thighs. Numerous diets, exercise and way of life suggestions address the question of the way excess frame fats can be efficaciously and completely reduced.

TIPS & TRICKS TO LOSE WEIGHT QUICKLY

➢ Drink plenty of water

Water is extremely important for our body as it is the prerequisite for many basic functions of our body. You should drink 2 to 3 liters of water a day. Sufficient fluids stimulate the body's metabolism and thus help you lose weight faster. In addition, water also helps against feeling hungry. It is best to drink half a liter of water before you eat and you will find that your feeling of hunger will subside faster as you eat. If you are not used to drinking so much water, water can quickly become boring. The taste of the water can be improved with many ingredients. Mint, ginger, cucumber or various berries are just a few ways to make the taste of the water more interesting.

➢ Refrain from alcohol

Most alcoholic beverages are not only high in calories, but also inhibit fat loss as the body is busy breaking down the alcohol. Above all, if you want to lose weight quickly, you should completely avoid alcohol while you are losing weight.

➢ Eat more vegetables

Most vegetables have very few calories in relation to their size and therefore fill you up faster due to the higher volume. A third of your daily meal should consist of vegetables. This not only helps you lose weight faster. It is also significantly healthier at the same time.

➢ Go for a walk

Anyone who wants to lose weight quickly needs a lot of exercise in everyday life. If you don't like doing sports, you can go for a walk regularly. Many calories are not burned when walking, but especially after eating, the walk stimulates the metabolism. In addition, walks reduce stress and clear your head, because losing weight is primarily a matter of the head.

➢ Fruit instead of candy

Food cravings are the biggest enemy of losing weight fast. Head and body crave sugar and the chocolate bar is suddenly very attractive again. It is often enough to give yourself some time and wait, because most food cravings will soon subside. If nothing else is possible, prefer the apple to the chocolate bar.

➢ Use stairs instead of elevator

If you want to lose weight quickly, you shouldn't miss any opportunity for exercise in everyday life. Take the stairs instead of the elevator and remember your goals every time. That also strengthens motivation.

➢ More protein instead of carbohydrates

Protein saturates significantly longer than carbohydrates, as the body has to use more energy for digestion. In addition, the body produces less insulin after the intake of protein, which is good for fat metabolism. In order to lose weight, the ratio of fat, protein and carbohydrates is not the only important factor. Be careful not to consume too many calories overall.

➢ Skipping a meal

It doesn't always have to be 3 meals. If you have a balanced diet and pay attention to your macronutrient distribution, two balanced meals should be enough. The two meals can also be placed in such a way that there is a break of around 14-18 hours between dinner and breakfast or lunch. If the body does not consume any food during this period, it slowly switches from burning glycogen (burning sugar) to metabolizing fat. That is the basic concept of intermittent fasting. If you want to lose weight quickly, you should try to get such a break in your diet.

Tip: By skipping a meal, you can easily increase the break between the last and the first meal and thus activate your fat metabolism. It is important, however, that you do not eat any food during the fasting hours. Even the milk in coffee is enough to slow down the fat metabolism again. Find out more about all intermittent fasting methods for losing weight and find the method that suits you.

➤ No sugary drinks

Many drinks contain significantly more sugar than we think. But what our body actually needs through drinks is liquid. If you want to lose weight quickly, you should completely switch to water.

➤ Sleep well and a lot

In sleep we regenerate and recharge our batteries for the next day. Those who have been well rested are more concentrated and more balanced. The willingness to be active during the day increases and a lot becomes easier. Also, the fight against food cravings. During restless sleep, the body also produces the appetite-stimulating hormone ghrelin, which promotes obesity.

➤ Use smaller plates

The size of the plate also affects our feeling of satiety. Studies on the subject of "influencing behavior through design" have shown that smaller plates unconsciously arouse the expectation in us that the food will fill us up much faster. Smaller plates can help you lose weight faster, but it should be clear that that won't work with the espresso saucer.

➤ No snacks

Snacks offer many ways to cheat. If you want to lose weight quickly, you have also decided to lose weight more radically. In a balanced diet with 2 to 3 meals there is unfortunately not much space left for snacks if you want to lose weight quickly. The only exception would be a lot of sport. After exercise, the body is particularly good at breaking down glucose and protein. It is best to plan your workout so that you also have your meal afterwards. If you're exercising on an empty stomach and your next meal is still a long way off, a post-workout snack is appropriate. Fruit is a great way to get your blood sugar back up after exercising.

➤ Avoid stress

Chronic stress in particular makes it difficult for you to lose weight. Stress causes the body to produce more of the stress hormone cortisol, which in turn slows down fat metabolism. Those who are balanced also make the many decisions about losing weight in everyday life much more rationally.

➢ Use bike instead of car

Another and often neglected way to bring more exercise into everyday life and thus lose weight faster is to get on the saddle instead of in the car. In addition, the bike is not only good for your figure, but also for the environment.

➢ Less carbohydrates in the evening

Carbohydrate-rich food increases blood sugar levels particularly quickly. As a result, more insulin is released, which is responsible for transporting blood sugar into the muscle cells. Since our muscle cells only work little or not at all in the evening and our body is set to rest, this energy is deposited in fat tissue. Of course, if you want to lose weight quickly, that's the last thing you want. If you eat less carbohydrates in the evening, you will lose weight faster.

➢ A quick workout in the morning

In the morning our carbohydrate stores are still empty and the body relies primarily on fat stores for its energy. A short and easy workout in the morning is therefore particularly effective for burning fat and losing weight faster. However, one should not overdo it. A too demanding workout on an empty stomach can quickly lead to lack of concentration and increase the risk of injury.

➢ Relax

Losing weight quickly means stress for the head above all. In addition to chocolate and fast food, you should also avoid mental stress, as otherwise there is a risk of cravings. Consciously take time for yourself to clear your head. That could be a wellness day in the thermal baths or a cozy afternoon on the sofa with a good book. Whatever helps you relax, do it.

➢ Go to the sauna

In the sauna, water is primarily removed, but regular use of the sauna can support the diet. The special conditions in the sauna promote the purification of the body through sweating and at the same time stimulate the fat metabolism. No one can lose weight quickly by going to the sauna alone, but the combination of a balanced diet, exercise and regular sauna bathing can accelerate weight loss.

➢ skipping rope

Jumping rope is one of the most effective workouts and can be very useful in helping you lose weight quickly. Various studies on the subject of "jumping rope" have shown that rope training is far more effective than jogging. This is largely due to the significantly higher muscle tone in the motion sequences. When jumping, the whole body has to work. The nice thing about it is: by concentrating on coordination, you notice the effort much less.

➢ Don't shop hungry

Hunger makes the shopping trolley full and then a few unhealthy things quickly end up in the trolley. By the way, researchers have also found that hunger when shopping does not only affect food consumption. The likelihood of buying other things, such as shoes, clothing or electrical appliances, increases when you go shopping.

➢ Drink coffee black

Those who like to drink coffee and want to lose weight quickly should only drink their coffee black. Coffee with milk, cappuccino or latte macchiato are quite the sugar traps, even without added sugar.

➢ Lots of tea

Tea is a very good alternative to coffee. Even without sugar, teas are an easy way to add variety to the diet. Although tea is not a magic potion and melts the fat, some types of tea have quite slimming properties that can help your diet to lose weight quickly. They boost the metabolism and calm the nerves. The classic slimming teas include green tea, ginger tea, mint tea, rooibos tea and mate tea.

➢ Cold showers

Cold showers remove heat and thus energy from the body. This is helpful when losing weight quickly, as the alternating bath not only strengthens the immune system, but also increases energy expenditure for a short time due to the heat extracted. The short overcoming of turning the tap to cold again at the end of the normal shower has many other advantages. Better blood circulation, improved sleep and faster regeneration after training are just some of the numerous advantages of contrast baths.

➢ Eat slower

It takes about 15-20 minutes for you to feel full. Anyone who gulps down their food during this time does not even give their body the opportunity to be full. This results in more calories being absorbed than would be the case with slower food. If you want to lose weight quickly, you should take your time while eating and enjoy it, after all, eating is something beautiful. In addition, chewing a lot helps with digestion, because it starts in the mouth. The saliva takes care of the decomposition of the carbohydrates in the mouth. By extensive chewing you also relieve your stomach and intestines.

➢ Hidden sugar

Sugar is a very popular ingredient in the food industry. So popular that many foods are secret sugar bombs. In addition to lemonades and juices, almost all sauces are sugar traps. A look at the list of ingredients often doesn't help, as the industry has come up with many cover names for the bad word. Dextrin, fructose, and glucose are just a few of the many new names for sugar. In order to lose weight faster and not fall for hidden sugars, the following rule of thumb applies: the more the food has been processed, the greater the likelihood that it will contain sugar.

➢ More fiber

Dietary fiber has a low energy density because it largely remains undigested. Thus, they fill you up earlier and help you lose weight quickly. Even if the name is a bit misleading, fiber is anything but ballast for the body. Soluble as well as insoluble fiber play a major role in the intestines and metabolism. Even if you do not want to lose weight, you should make sure that you have a sufficient intake of fiber. The DGE recommends at least 30 grams of fiber per day. Foods high in fiber include whole grains, vegetables, legumes, potatoes, nuts, and seeds.

➢ Throwing unhealthy food out of your home

Many have a place in their home where they can escape from food cravings. If you want to lose weight quickly but still have 10 kilos of chocolate in the house, it won't be easier for you. You make it easier for yourself if you don't have unhealthy foods around when you diet. Provide healthy alternatives such as tea or fruit.

➢ HIIT workout

Interval training is an intense workout that quickly shows results. Intensive intervals alternate with short active breaks. These are designed in such a way that the organism cannot fully recover, which creates a strong training stimulus. The maximum oxygen uptake creates a certain afterburn effect, which also ensures an increased calorie consumption after training. This in turn helps to lose weight faster. However, the prerequisite is that you go to your limits during training. If you don't sweat here, you're doing something wrong.

➢ Fixed dates for sports

Especially those who don't like sports find it difficult to train regularly. If you find it difficult to get yourself up for training, you should plan your sport with fixed dates. Fixed times help develop routines. This can be, for example, a sporting date with a friend. Fixed courses in fitness studios are also good for your own routines in sports. If you want to lose weight quickly, you can support rapid weight loss through regular and effective training.

> ➤ **Chewing gum for cravings**

You should be prepared for food cravings. If a cup of tea or a walk doesn't help, sugar-free gum can satisfy those cravings. Chewing gum can satisfy the desire to chew and thus help those with a sweet tooth to lose weight faster.

HERE ARE 10 BENEFITS OF WEIGHT LOSS AND TIPS FOR DOING IT SAFELY.

1. Helps regulate blood sugar and diabetes

Losing weight improves insulin sensitivity in people with type 2 diabetes, says Preeti Pusalkar, a certified clinical nutritionist at Hudson Medical Center, a primary care facility in New York City, United States.

The excess body fat leads to increased adipose tissue, causing inflammation and interferes with the function of insulin, the hormone that helps to regulate the levels of blood sugar.

Losing a few pounds helps to reduce this adipose tissue, allowing the body to manage blood sugar more effectively.

Plus, you don't need to lose weight dramatically to see results. The investigations have found that only a reduction of 5% of body weight in adulthood, improves these sugar levels.

2. Improve your heart health

Reduce some kilos can also improve the health of the heart to the lower pressure in the arteries, which means that the heart does not have to work so hard to pump blood throughout the body.

The result is lower blood pressure and levels of low-density lipoprotein (LDL) cholesterol, the "bad" type of cholesterol that can increase the risk of heart disease, Pusalkar specifies.

For more, it doesn't even depend on how you lose weight.

Whether you lose weight by changing your diet and exercising, or if you undergo an operation to lose weight such as metabolic surgery, you will also obtain benefits, according to a study published in 2020.

The researchers examined the effects of weight loss surgery in obese patients who underwent it or who lost weight through lifestyle changes.

The risk of heart disease for the group that underwent the operation decreased after a loss of between 5% and 10% of body weight, while the non-surgical group saw a decrease after losing about 20% of the body weight.

3. Decreases the risk of strokes

The excess kilograms in your body can increase blood pressure. Hence, also the risk of having a stroke.

This is because high blood pressure puts stress on the blood vessels, making them stiffer and more likely to cause blood to clot.

"Losing weight helps improve the efficiency of the heart because the blood vessels are less constricted," says Pusalkar.

4. You sleep better

Overweight people are more likely to suffer from sleep apnea, a disorder characterized by the interruption of breathing during sleep.

This is because being overweight can increase fat deposits in the neck, which could block the airways.

If you suffer from sleep apnea, losing weight probably won't completely cure the condition.

However, losing just 10 to 15% of your body weight can improve sleep quality and reduce the severity of sleep apnea in moderately obese patients, according to the US National Sleep Foundation.

5. Improve your mobility

Lowering your body weight relieves pressure on your knees and joints, which tends to improve mobility, Pusalkar notes.

A 2012 study of obese adults with type 2 diabetes found that just a 1% decrease in weight reduced mobility limitations, such as difficulty walking or climbing stairs, by more than 7%.

6. Raise your self-esteem

While there is no direct correlation between losing weight and self-esteem, some studies show that losing weight can improve mood and self-confidence.

In a 2014 review, 36 studies were examined to determine the psychological benefits of weight loss. The researchers found consistent improvements in body image, self-esteem, and general well-being among the subjects who lost weight.

7. Decrease in joint pain

Excess weight can cause joints to become tight, damaged, and inflamed. But losing those extra pounds can help you improve it.

A study conducted in 2018 examined obese adults with arthritic knee pain.

The researchers found that losing 10% to 20% of body weight resulted in less pain and improved joint function than losing just 5% of body weight, which showed no significant benefit to the body. joint pain

The reason probably has to do with how quickly the joints wear out when they are under additional stress from excess weight.

"As the smooth surface at the ends of the bones, or cartilage, becomes damaged and wears down, you feel pain and stiffness in the joint," explains Pulsalkar.

8. Increase your energy

As much as it improves your hours and quality of sleep, your energy during the day can also be benefited, highlights Pulsalkar.

Meanwhile, excess weight also means that your body has to work harder to move. Therefore, losing a few pounds means that you will use less energy to move.

In turn, this will improve your respiratory function by encouraging you to feel more energetic.

9. Increase your sexual desire

Research on the correlation between excess weight and sexual desire is still in the making.

But others have shown that weight gain increases the levels of sex hormone-linked globulin (SHBG) in the blood. This would lead to a reduction in free testosterone levels and a decrease in libido, explains Pulsalkar.

10. Reduces the risk of certain types of cancer

According to the American Cancer Society, excess body weight is the cause of about 11% of cancer cases in women and about 5% in men.

Obesity increases the risk of developing several different cancers, including:

- Endometrial cancer
- Breast cancer (in women who have gone through menopause)
- Kidney cancer
- Liver cancer
- Pancreatic cancer

The exact relationship between excess weight and cancer is still unknown, but researchers believe that inflammation due to visceral fat - the fat that surrounds vital organs - is to blame.

However, some people may need to lose a lot more weight to experience some of these benefits,

But, for most, losing as little as 5% of your body weight can yield many health benefits, such as better heart health and a lower risk of diabetes.

However, before starting any weight loss program, it is important that you consult with a specialist about the plan and goals that are right for you.

WEIGHT LOSS RECIPES
Salad with chicken strips

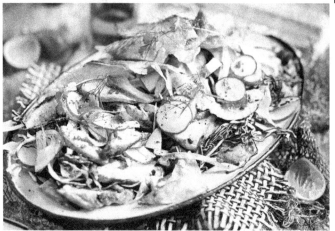

Ingredients For 4 people

- 1 red chilli pepper
- 1 clove of garlic
- 6 tbsp olive oil
- 4 tbsp Lime juice
- Salt, pepper, mexican
- 1 tsp Liquid honey
- fennel
- 1 federal government radish
- 200 g Red cabbage
- 1 Red onion
- 1 avocado
- 1 Tortillas (wraps)
- 500 g Chicken fillets
- 4 stems parsley

preparation

40 minutes

1. Clean, cut lengthways, core and wash the chilli pepper. Peel the garlic and finely chop it with the chilli. Mix 4 tablespoons of oil, lime juice, chilli and garlic. Season to taste with salt and honey.

2. Clean the fennel, put the greens aside and wash both. Clean and wash the radishes and red cabbage. Peel the onion. Plan or cut everything into fine slices. Halve the avocado, remove the stone, remove the pulp from the skin and cut into slices. Mix the prepared ingredients and the chilli dressing. To taste.

3. Cut the tortillas into strips. Wash the chicken, pat dry, season with salt. Heat 1 tablespoon of oil in a pan, toast the tortillas for about 3 minutes while turning until crispy. Take out, add 1 tablespoon of oil to the hot pan and fry the chicken fillets for about 5 minutes on each side. Season with Mexican spice mixture.

4. Wash the parsley and shake dry. Cut the chicken fillets into strips. Arrange the salad with the chicken and the crispy tortilla strips. Sprinkle with parsley and the chopped fennel leaves.

Nutritional info

1 portion approx:

400 kcal33 g protein22 g fat14 g of carbohydrates

Crazy delicious cauliflower soup

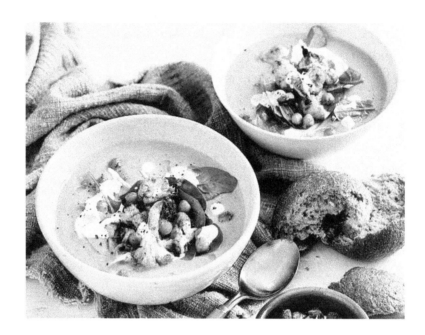

Ingredients For 4 people

- 2 cans (425 ml each) Chickpeas
- 1 large cauliflower
- 6 tbsp olive oil
- Curry powder, ground coriander, salt, pepper
- 1 tsp Vegetable broth (instant)
- 50 g Baby spinach
- 1 lemon
- 150 g Greek yogurt (10% fat)
- Parchment paper

preparation

50 minutes

1   Preheat the oven (electric stove: 200 ° C / convection: 180 ° C / gas: see manufacturer). Line a tray with baking paper. Drain the chickpeas. Clean the cauliflower, cut into florets, wash. Mix both with oil, 3 tablespoons of curry and 1⁄2 teaspoon each of coriander, salt and pepper. Spread on the baking sheet and bake in the oven for about 25–30 minutes.

2   Set aside about 1⁄4 of the cauliflower and chickpea mix. Bring the rest to the boil with 1 1⁄2 l of water in a large saucepan, stir in the stock. Cover the soup and simmer for about 5 minutes.

3   Sort the spinach, wash and shake dry. Puree the soup finely. Season to taste with salt, pepper and the lemon juice. Briefly heat the rest of the cauliflower mix in the soup. Serve with yogurt and spinach.

Nutritional info

1 portion approx:

270 kcal9 g protein20 g fat12 g of carbohydrates

Relaxed medallions with sweet and spicy sauce

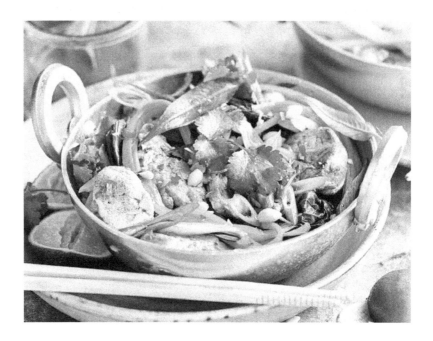

Ingredients For 4 people

- 1 piece (approx. 2 cm each) ginger
- 600 g pork tenderloin
- 400 g Baby Pak Choi
- 400 g Carrots
- 2 Spring onions
- 1 red chilli pepper
- 2 tbsp Soy sauce
- 1-2 tsp Liquid honey
- 8-10 stems Asian herbs (e.g. coriander, Vietnamese mint or Thai basil)
- 2-3 tbsp oil
- salt
- 6 tbsp roasted, salted peanuts

preparation

40 minutes

1. Peel the ginger and grate finely. Squeeze the limes. Pat the pork tenderloin dry and cut into medallions. Mix with ginger and 4 tbsp lime juice, marinate for about 15 minutes.
2. In the meantime, clean and wash the Pak Choi and cut into strips. Peel and wash the carrots and cut lengthways into strips. Clean and wash the spring onions and cut diagonally into rings.
3. For the sauce, clean the chilli, cut lengthways, core, wash and finely chop. Mix the rest of the lime juice, chilli, soy sauce, honey and 3 tablespoons of water. Wash herbs, shake dry, pluck leaves.
4. Heat oil in a large pan. Fry the meat in portions for 1–2 minutes on each side. Salt and take out. Add the carrots, pak choi and 2 tablespoons of water to the pan and cook for about 3 minutes. Sauté the spring onions and meat for 1 minute. Season to taste with salt. Arrange the vegetables and meat, sprinkle with nuts and herbs. Drizzle with sauce.

Nutritional info

1 portion approx:

380 kcal41 g protein17 g fat12 g of carbohydrates

A quick salad with lentils

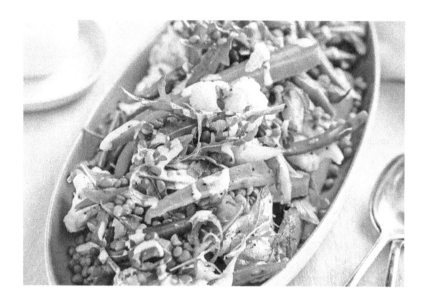

Ingredients For 4 people

- 4th Carrots
- 1 cauliflower
- salt and pepper
- 200 g green beans
- 2 cans Lentils (425 ml each)
- 75 g arugula
- 1 clove of garlic
- 3 tbsp Tahini (sesame paste; glass)
- 1-2 tsp Maple syrup
- 4 tbsp Lemon juice
- 2 tbsp olive oil

preparation

30 minutes

Peel and wash the carrots and quarter them lengthways. Clean the cauliflower, cut into florets and wash. Cook the vegetables in a large saucepan in salted water for about 8-10 minutes. In the meantime, clean and wash the beans, cut in half lengthways and cook for the last 4 minutes. Drain the vegetables, rinse in cold water and let them drain.

In the meantime, rinse the lentils in the sieve and let them drain well. Sort out the rocket, wash and shake dry.

Peel and finely chop the clove of garlic. Mix with tahini, maple syrup, lemon juice, oil and approx. 4 tablespoons of water to make a salad sauce, season with salt and pepper. Mix the prepared ingredients, serve and drizzle with the tahini salad sauce.

Nutritional info

1 portion approx:

240 kcal11 g protein11 g fat22 g of carbohydrates

Veggie bowl with fried egg

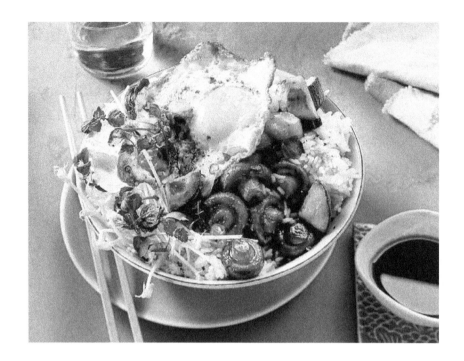

Ingredients For 4 people

- 400 g Champingons
- 1 zucchini
- 200 g Long grain rice
- salt
- 3-4 tbsp olive oil
- 4 tbsp Soy sauce
- 2 tbsp Sriracha sauce (hot chili sauce)
- 1 tbsp sesame oil
- 50 g Pea or mung bean sprouts
- 1-2 red chili peppers
- 4th Eggs
- 1 box red shiso cress

preparation

35 minutes

1   Clean the mushrooms and wash them if necessary. Clean and wash the zucchini, quarter lengthways, cut into pieces. Prepare rice in approx. 400 ml boiling salted water according to the instructions on the packet.

2   In the meantime, heat 2–3 tablespoons of oil in a large pan. Fry the mushrooms in it. Add zucchini and fry for about 4 minutes. Stir in soy and sriracha sauce, sesame oil and 3 tablespoons of water, briefly bring to the boil. Take off the stove and keep warm.
3   Sort the sprouts, rinse and drain. Clean and wash the chilli and cut into rings with the seeds. Heat 1 tablespoon of oil in another pan. Fry eggs with fried eggs, season with salt. Cut the cress from the bed. Arrange rice and vegetables in bowls. Spread the fried eggs and sprouts on top, sprinkle with cress. Scatter chilli on top as desired.

Nutritional info

1 portion approx:

400 kcal16 g protein17 g fat44 g of carbohydrates

Stuffed peppers "Spicy Renner"

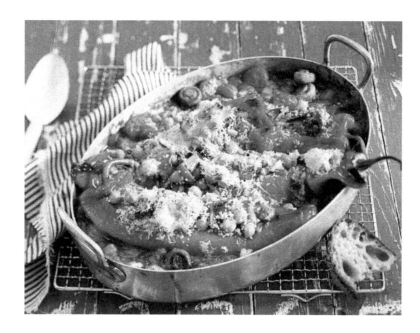

Ingredients For 4 people

- 3 Spring onions
- 125 g couscous
- 1/2 tsp Vegetable broth (instant)
- 2 can (s) (425 ml each) chunky tomatoes
- 1 can (s) (425 ml each) Chickpeas
- 250 g Cherry tomatoes
- 150 g small mushrooms
- Salt, pepper, sugar, dried oregano
- 1 tsp Sambal Oelek
- 4th red pointed pepper (approx. 150 g each)
- 2 tbsp Lemon juice
- 2 tbsp olive oil
- 75 g Parmesan or vegetarian hard cheese (piece)

preparation

20 minutes (+ 30 minutes waiting time)

1 Preheat the oven (electric stove: 200 ° C / convection: 180 ° C / gas: see manufacturer). Bring 175 ml of water to the boil. Clean and wash the spring onions, cut into rings. Mix the couscous and broth in a bowl, top with the spring onions. Pour boiling water over the couscous mix, cover and leave to soak for approx. 5 minutes.

2   Rinse and drain the chickpeas. Wash the cherry tomatoes and cut in half. Clean the mushrooms. Put half of the chickpeas, cherry tomatoes and mushrooms with chunky tomatoes in a baking dish. Season with salt, pepper, 1 teaspoon sugar, 2 teaspoons oregano and sambal oelek. Put in the oven.

3   Cut a rectangle lengthways from each pepper and dice it into small pieces. Core and wash the peppers. Add the diced paprika, lemon juice, oil and the rest of the chickpeas to the couscous, mix. Season with salt and pepper and pour into the peppers.

4   Place the stuffed peppers on top of the vegetables. Grate the cheese finely. Bake in the hot oven for about 30 minutes.

Nutritional info

1 portion approx:

390 kcal15 g protein16 g fat44 g of carbohydrates

Fillet with pak choi

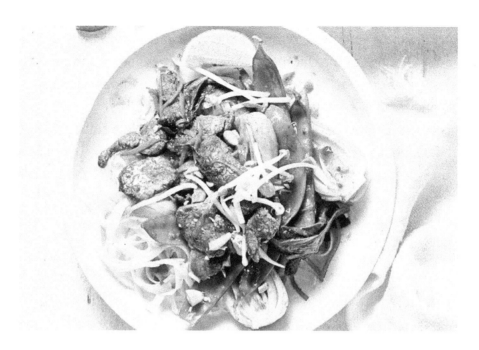

Ingredients For 4 people

- 400 g pork tenderloin
- spice powder
- 3 tbsp Almonds (skinless)
- 1 carrot
- 2 Garlic cloves
- 1 piece (approx. 2 cm) ginger
- 500 g Baby Pak Choi
- 100 g sugar snap
- 75 g Mung bean sprouts
- 2-3 tbsp oil
- 3 tbsp Lime juice
- 6 tbsp Soy sauce
- 2 tbsp sweet chili sauce

preparation

30 minutes

1   Pat the fillet dry, cut into thin slices and mix with 1 teaspoon of 5-spice powder. Chop the almonds. Peel and wash the carrot and cut into fine strips. Peel and chop the garlic and ginger. Clean and wash the pak choi, cut in half lengthways. Clean and wash snow peas. Sort out the sprouts, wash them and let them drain.

2   Heat oil in a large pan. Fry the fillet in portions over high heat, remove. Sauté the carrots, garlic and ginger in the hot frying fat. Add the pak choi, lime juice, 2 tbsp water, soy and chili sauce, bring to the boil, continue cooking for approx. 2 minutes. Fold in the fillet and sugar snap peas, heat for approx. 1 minute. Sprinkle with the almonds and sprouts. Rice noodles also taste good.

Nutritional info

1 portion approx:

280 kcal29 g protein13 g fat9 g of carbohydrates

Salmon on Spinach Salad

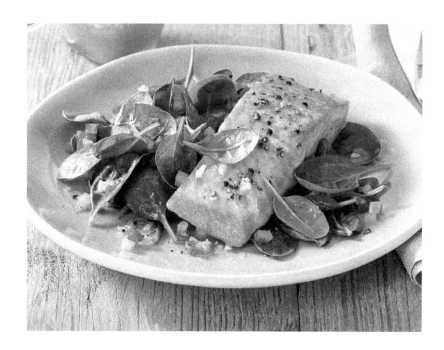

Ingredients For 4 people

- 1 Organic lime
- 10 g fresh ginger
- 1 Shallot
- Juice of 1 orange
- salt
- pepper from the grinder
- 100 g Baby spinach leaves
- red and yellow pepper
- 4th Salmon fillets (approx. 160 g each)
- 50 g Flour
- 2 tbsp olive oil

preparation

25 minutes

1   Wash the lime with hot water, rub dry, finely grate the peel and squeeze out the juice. Peel the ginger and grate finely. Peel and finely dice shallot. Mix the ginger, shallot, orange juice, lime juice and zest together. Season to taste with salt and pepper. Clean and wash the spinach and spin dry. Halve the peppers, clean, wash and cut into fine cubes

2   Rinse fillets with cold water, pat dry, season with salt and pepper. Put the flour on a flat plate. Turn the fillets in it. Heat oil in a large pan. Fry fillets over medium heat for 2-3 minutes on each side
3   Mix the spinach, paprika and dressing and arrange on plates with the salmon fillets

Nutritional info

1 person approx:

400 kcal1680 kJ34 g protein25 g fat9 g of carbohydrates

Turnip curry with steak involtini

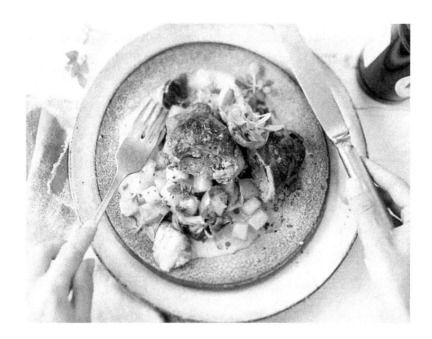

Ingredients For 4 people

- 800 g Turnip
- Salt, pepper, curry
- 5 stems oregano
- 5 stems basil
- onion
- 500 g Hoof steak
- 1vtsp medium hot mustard
- 3 tbsp oil
- 1 piece (approx. 4 cm each) ginger
- 1 red chilli pepper
- 3 Shallots
- 1 can (s) (400 ml each) unsweetened coconut milk
- 1 tbsp food starch
- 200 g Brussels sprouts

preparation

60 minutes

1   Peel and wash the turnip and cut into 1 cm cubes. Cook in salted boiling water for 5–7 minutes. Drain, collecting approx. 200 ml of the cooking water.

2   For the involtini, wash the herbs, shake dry and roughly chop the stems. Peel and finely dice the onion. Preheat the oven (electric stove: 100 ° C / convection: 80 ° C / gas: not

suitable). Pat the meat dry and cut into 4 slices. Knock between 2 layers of foil thinner. Brush the meat with mustard. Spread the onion and herbs on top, roll up.

3   Heat 2 tablespoons of oil in a large pan. Fry the involtini vigorously all around. Season with salt and pepper, cook on a tray in the hot oven for about 25 minutes. Set aside the pan with the frying fat.

4   For the curry, peel and finely chop the ginger. Clean the chilli, cut lengthways, core, wash and chop very finely. Peel and finely dice shallots. Heat 1 tablespoon of oil in a saucepan. Briefly sauté the ginger, chilli and shallots in it. Dust with 1 teaspoon of curry and sauté briefly. Deglaze with the cooking water and coconut milk, bring to the boil. Add the turnip, simmer for about 2 minutes. Mix the starch and 2 tbsp water until smooth, use it to thicken the curry. Season to taste with salt and pepper.

5   Clean the Brussels sprouts, cut off the stalk generously, wash and press down with the heel of your hand so that the individual leaves come off. Reheat the pan with the frying fat. Fry the Brussels sprouts in it for 2-3 minutes. Season with salt and pepper. Serve with curry and involtini.

Nutritional info

1 portion approx:

400 kcal35 g protein20 g fat17 g of carbohydrates

Baked sweet potato

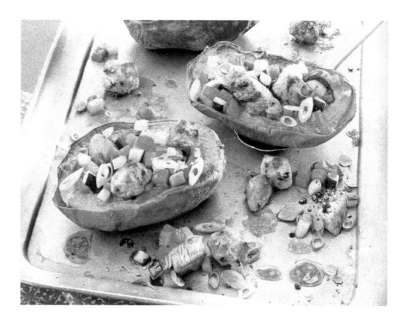

Ingredients For 4 people

- 2 big sweet potatoes
- 2 red and yellow pepper
- zucchini
- 300 g Chicken fillet
- 2 tbsp oil
- salt
- pepper
- 3 Spring onions
- Parchment paper
- 5 tbsp homemade barbecue sauce

For the barbecue sauce

- 2 Onions
- 2 tbsp Coconut oil
- 1 tsp Tomato paste
- 1 can (s) (425 ml) sieved tomatos
- 250 ml Vegetable broth
- 100 ml Apple Cider Vinegar
- 5 tbsp honey
- 1 tsp pepper
- 1 tsp mustard
- 1 tsp smoked paprika powder

- 1 tbsp Lime juice
- salt

preparation

45 minutes

1. Wash the potatoes and cut in half lengthways. Place the potatoes with the cut side up on a baking sheet lined with baking paper and bake in the preheated oven (electric stove: 175 ° C / convection: 150 ° C / gas: see manufacturer) for about 45 minutes.
2. For the barbecue sauce, peel and finely dice the onions. Heat oil in a pot. Sauté the onions in it. Add tomato paste and fry for about 3 minutes. Add the remaining ingredients and stir.
3. Let simmer for about 1 hour, stirring occasionally. Season with salt and let cool.
4. Clean and wash the peppers and zucchini and cut into cubes. Wash the meat, pat dry and cut into approx. 2 cm cubes. Heat the oil in a pan and fry the meat for about 5 minutes, turning.
5. Season with salt and pepper. Take out and keep warm. Sauté the paprika and zucchini in the frying fat. Also season with salt and pepper.
6. Clean and wash the spring onions and cut diagonally into rings. Take the potatoes out of the oven and let them cool down a little. Hollow out about 1/3 of the potato with a tablespoon. Mix the meat and vegetables.
7. Season with barbecue sauce and spread over the potatoes. Sprinkle with spring onions.

Nutritional info

1 person approx:

340 kcal1420 kJ21 g protein7 g fat47 g of carbohydrates

Zucchini salad with broccoli pesto

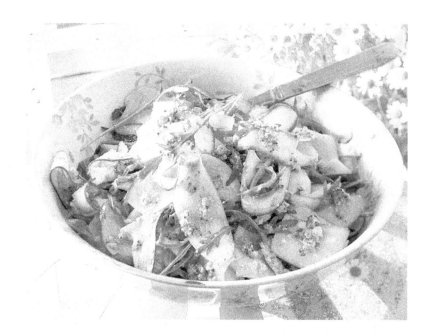

Ingredients For 6 people

- 2 Zucchini (approx. 400 g; e.g. green and yellow)
- 1 (approx. 60 g) large bunch of rocket
- 500 g broccoli
- Salt pepper
- 2 Garlic cloves
- 50 g Skinless almond kernels
- 50 g Parmesan or vegetarian hard cheese (piece)
- 100 ml good olive oil

preparation

35 minutes

1 Clean and wash the zucchini and slice lengthways into wafer-thin slices with a peeler or with a slicer. Clean, wash and roughly cut the rocket. Mix the zucchini and rocket in a bowl.

2 Clean and wash broccoli and cut into small florets. Cook the broccoli in a little salted boiling water for about 2 minutes. Drain the broccoli and place in a tall mixing bowl.

3 Peel and roughly chop the garlic. Chop the almonds. Grate the parmesan. Add the garlic, almonds and parmesan to the broccoli. Coarsely puree everything with a hand blender. Pour in the oil, continuing to purée. Season well with salt and pepper.

4 Pour the broccoli pesto over the zucchini salad and mix everything together. Season the salad with salt and pepper.

Nutritional info

1 person approx:

260 kcal7 g protein24 g fat3 g of carbohydrates

Beguiling lentil soup "magic ginger"

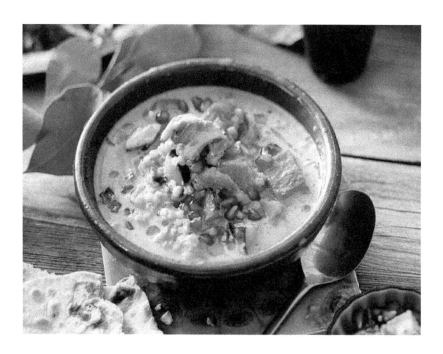

Ingredients For 6 people

- 1 Hokkaido pumpkin (approx. 1.2 kg each)
- 2 Zucchini (approx. 250 g each)
- 2 Onions
- 3 Garlic cloves
- 1 piece (approx. 4 cm each) ginger
- 3 tbsp oil
- 300 g yellow lentils (alternatively red lentils)
- Curry powder, salt, pepper
- 2 tbsp Agave syrup
- 3 tsp Vegetable broth (instant)
- 2 Bay leaves
- 400 g Cherry tomatoes
- pomegranate
- Avocados
- Limes
- 150 g Greek cream yogurt

preparation

50 minutes

1. Wash the pumpkin, cut in half, remove the seeds and soft fibers. Cut the pumpkin into cubes. Wash, clean and dice the zucchini. Peel and finely dice onions, garlic and ginger.
2. Heat the oil in a large saucepan. Sauté onions, garlic and ginger in it. Add the pumpkin and zucchini, fry for about 5 minutes. Rinse, drain and add the lentils. Dust with 1 tbsp curry and sweat. Pour in 1.4 l of water and agave syrup, bring to the boil. Stir in the vegetable stock, add the bay leaf. Season with salt and pepper. Cover and simmer for about 20 minutes.
3. Wash and quarter the cherry tomatoes. Halve the pomegranate and remove the seeds. Halve and core the avocados. Remove the pulp from the skin with a tablespoon and cut into small pieces. Drizzle with half of the lime juice.
4. Puree some of the soup as desired. Heat the tomatoes in the soup. Season to taste with salt, pepper and the rest of the lime juice. Stir in yogurt (do not boil anymore!). Serve with avocado pieces and pomegranate seeds.

Nutritional info

1 portion approx:

250 kcal13 g protein10 g fat28 g of carbohydrates

Kohlrabi schnitzel with yogurt and herb dip

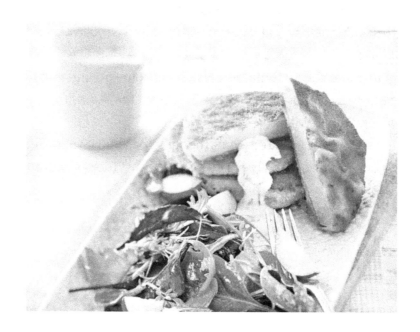

Ingredients For 4 people

- 800 g Kohlrabi
- salt
- pepper
- 2 Eggs (size M)
- tbsp Flour
- 80 g breadcrumbs
- tbsp oil
- 1/2 bunch chives
- 6 stem (s) parsley
- Bed of cress
- 150 g Whole milk yogurt
- Splash of lemon juice
- sugar
- 3 tbsp Fruit vinegar
- 1 tsp honey
- 1/2 bunch radish
- 200 g Baby leaf salad mix

preparation

35 minutes

1. Peel the kohlrabi and cut into approx. 1.5 cm thick slices. Season with salt and pepper. Whisk eggs. Turn kohlrabi slices first in flour, then in egg, then in breadcrumbs. Heat 2 tablespoons of oil in a large pan. Fry the kohlrabi in portions, turning, for about 6 minutes

2. Wash herbs, shake dry. Cut the chives into small rolls. Pluck the parsley leaves and chop finely. Cut about 2/3 of the cress from the bed. Stir the herbs into the yogurt. Season to taste with lemon juice, sugar, salt and pepper

3. For the vinaigrette, whisk together vinegar, salt, pepper and honey. Beat in 2 tablespoons of oil drop by drop. Clean, wash and quarter the radishes. Wash the lettuce and drain well in a colander. Mix the lettuce, radishes and vinaigrette together. Arrange 3 kohlrabi schnitzel, salad and yogurt dip on 4 plates. Cut the rest of the cress from the bed and sprinkle over the salad

Nutritional info

1 person approx:

290 kcal1210 kJ11 g protein15 g fat28 g of carbohydrates

Vegetable noodles with Bolognese

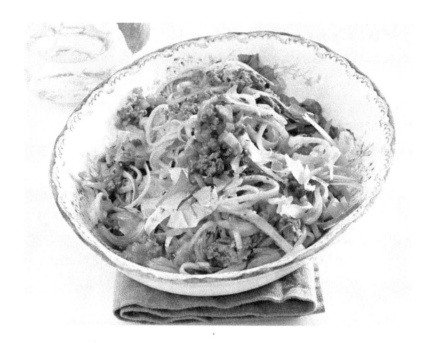

Ingredients For 4 people

- 1.5 kg small zucchini (e.g. green and yellow)
- 600 g Carrots
- 1 small bunch of soup greens
- 1 onion
- 1 tbsp olive oil
- 250 g Beefsteakhack
- Salt pepper
- 2 tbsp Tomato paste
- 1 tbsp Flour
- 1 tsp Vegetable broth (instant)
- 40 g Pecorino or Parmesan
- 1 small pot of basil

preparation

45 minutes

1   Clean or peel and wash the zucchini and carrots. Use a large, sharp knife to cut
    lengthways into thin slices, then into long, fine strips. Clean or peel the soup greens,

wash and cut into very small cubes. Peel onion and chop finely.

2   For the Bolognese, heat the oil in a large pan. Fry the mince in it until crumbly. Season with salt and pepper. Briefly sauté the prepared vegetable and onion cubes. Stir in tomato paste. Dust the flour over it and sauté briefly. Pour 400 ml of water and stir in the vegetable stock. Bring everything to the boil, simmer for 7–8 minutes.

3   In the meantime, cook the vegetable strips in plenty of salted boiling water for 3–5 minutes. Drain, collecting some of the cooking water. Put the vegetable strips for the Bolognese in the pan and mix everything well. If the sauce is not liquid enough, stir in some vegetable boiling water and season everything again.

4   Slice the cheese into fine shavings. Wash the basil, shake dry, pluck the leaves off and cut roughly. Arrange the vegetable noodles, sprinkle with parmesan and basil.

Nutritional info

1 person approx:

290 kcal26 g protein10 g fat21 g of carbohydrates

Giggle-giggle-chickpea stew

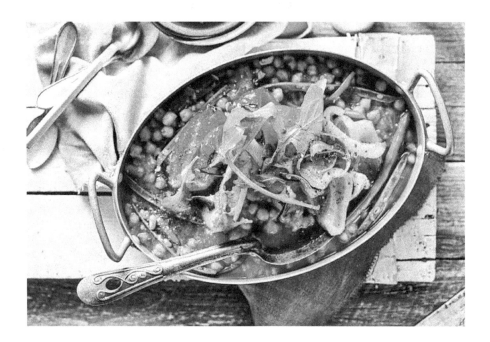

- ***Ingredients For 4 people***
- 350 g green beans (fresh or frozen)
- Salt, sweet paprika, pepper, sugar
- 2 can (s) (425 ml each) Chickpeas
- 200 g Mini peppers
- 2 Onions (e.g. red)
- 2 Garlic cloves
- 3tbsp olive oil
- 1 Cinnamon stick
- 1 can (s) (850 ml each) tomatoes
- some rocket

preparation

40 minutes

1   Clean the beans, wash them and cook them in salted water for about 8 minutes. Pour off, put off. Rinse and drain the chickpeas. Halve, core and wash the bell pepper. Peel and finely dice the onions and garlic.

2   Heat the oil in the pan. Sauté onions and garlic in it. Briefly sauté paprika and 3 teaspoons paprika powder. Add the chickpeas, cinnamon stick, tomatoes and 1⁄4 l

water, chop the tomatoes a little, bring to the boil. Season with salt, pepper and sugar. Simmer uncovered for 5–7 minutes until thick. Season again to taste. Heat the beans in it. Sprinkle with rocket if you like. In addition: baguette.

Nutritional info

1 portion approx:

350 kcal14 g protein13 g fat41 g of carbohydrates

Cauliflower curry with chicken breast

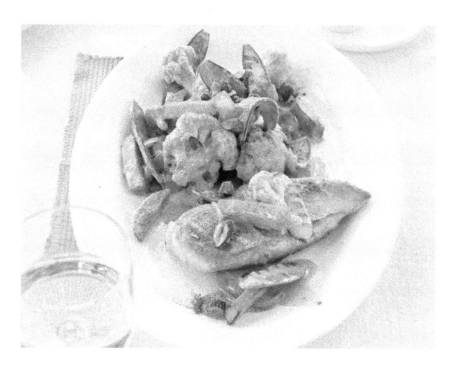

Ingredients For 2 people

- 300 g Carrots
- 1 Head of cauliflower
- salt
- 150 g sugar snap
- 1 small onion
- 1 clove of garlic
- 1 tbsp Sunflower oil
- 20 g Almond kernels with skin
- 2 (approx. 250 g) small chicken fillets
- 1-2 tbsp Madras curry powder
- 1 tsp Flour
- 100 g milk

preparation

40 minutes

1. Peel and wash the carrots and cut into sticks. Clean the cauliflower, cut into florets from the stem and wash. Blanch the carrots and cauliflower in boiling salted water for about 4 minutes. Wash and clean the sugar snap peas. Peel and dice the onion and garlic
2. Heat the oil in a pan and roast the almonds in it for about 4 minutes, turning. Wash the meat, pat dry and season with salt. Remove the almonds and fry the meat in the nut fat for about 8 minutes, turning
3. Take out the meat and keep it warm. Fry the onion and garlic in the frying fat for about 5 minutes. After about 2 minutes add the snow peas and drained cauliflower and carrots. Dust with curry and flour and roast for 1 more minute. Add milk, bring to the boil and simmer for about 2 minutes. Roughly chop the nuts. Arrange the curry and meat. Sprinkle with nuts

Nutritional info

1 person approx:

400 kcal1680 kJ41 g protein14 g fat25 g of carbohydrates

Cauliflower Rice

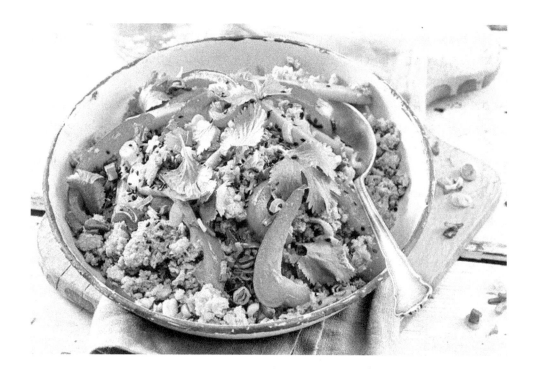

Ingredients For 4 people

- 800 g cauliflower
- 20 g fresh ginger
- 2 red peppers
- 2 Carrots
- 4th Spring onions
- stems coriander
- 3 tbsp sesame oil
- 3 tbsp Soy sauce
- Salt pepper
- 1 tsp Curry powder
- 4th Eggs (size M)
- 1 tbsp black sesame seeds

preparation

50 minutes

1   Clean the cauliflower, cut from the stalk in large florets and wash. Roughly grate the florets on a grater. Peel and finely dice the ginger. Wash and clean the peppers and cut into strips. Peel the carrots and cut into sticks. Wash and clean the spring onions and cut into fine rings. Wash the coriander, shake dry and pluck the leaves from the stems.

2   Heat 2 tablespoons of sesame oil in a large pan or wok. Fry the cauliflower rice in it for 3 -5 minutes while stirring. Add the ginger and deglaze with the soy sauce. Season with salt, pepper and curry powder. Heat 1 tablespoon of sesame oil in another pan, fry the paprika strips and carrot sticks for 3-5 minutes. Season with salt and pepper.

3   Whisk the eggs and pour over the cauliflower rice. Let the egg set while stirring. Add paprika, carrot and spring onion. Season to taste and serve in bowls. Garnish with coriander leaves and black sesame seeds and serve.

Nutritional info

1 portion approx:

280 kcal14 g protein16 g fat16 g of carbohydrates

Fried egg pan with gratin

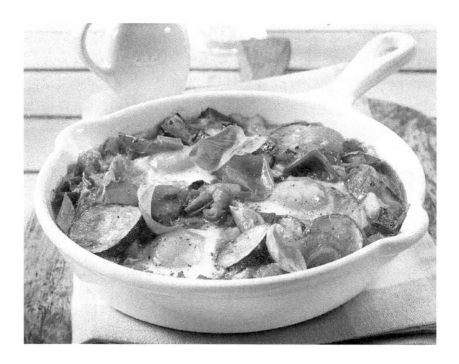

Ingredients For 4 people

- 2 Spring onions
- 1-2 Garlic cloves
- 600 g tomatoes
- 1 (approx. 400 g) aubergine
- (approx. 400 g) zucchini
- stem (s) basil
- 3-4 tbsp olive oil
- salt
- black pepper
- dried herbs of Provence
- 1-2 tbsp Tomato paste
- 2 tbsp dark balsamic vinegar
- 200 ml Vegetable broth
- sugar
- 4th Eggs (size M)

preparation

30 minutes

1   Wash and clean the spring onions. Dice the spring onion white, cut the spring onion greens into rings. Peel garlic and chop finely. Wash, clean and cut tomatoes, aubergines

and zucchini.

2   Wash the basil, pat dry and cut into strips except for something to garnish. Heat the olive oil in a large, non-stick pan with a high rim. Fry the aubergine and zucchini in it and season with salt, pepper and herbs from Provence.

3   Add spring onion and garlic and fry briefly. Add tomato paste and sauté briefly. Add tomatoes, vinegar, broth and basil and cook covered for 6–8 minutes. Season the ratatouille with salt, pepper and sugar.

4   Press 4 deep hollows into the ratatouille with a tablespoon. Carefully slide 1 egg each into the hollow. Cover the pan with a lid and let the eggs set over low heat for about 6 minutes.

5   Garnish with basil.

Nutritional info

1 person approx:

230 kcal960 kJ12 g protein15 g fat10 g of carbohydrates

Millet patties with lamb's lettuce and radish

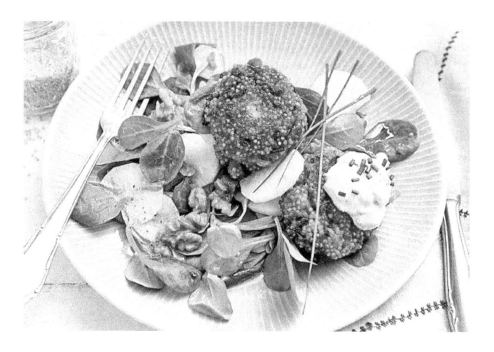

Ingredients For 4 people

- 200 g millet
- Salt pepper
- 1 onion
- 1 clove of garlic
- 150 g Beetroot (cooked, vacuum packed)
- 500 g radish
- 150 g Lamb's lettuce
- 1 federal government chives
- 250 g lowfat quark
- 3 tsp sweet mustard
- 1 tbsp Flour
- 2 tbsp Walnut kernels
- 2 tbsp oil
- 3 tbsp Apple Cider Vinegar

preparation

40 minutes

1   Rinse the millet. Bring 500 ml of salt water to the boil. Stir in millet. Let it soak for approx. 15 minutes with the stove switched off. Peel and finely dice the onion and

garlic. Roughly grate the beetroot. Clean and peel the radish. Cut about 2⁄3 into thin slices, coarsely grate the rest. Wash and clean the salad.

2   For the dip, wash the chives and cut into rolls. Mix the quark, 1 teaspoon mustard, grated radish and chives. Season with salt and pepper.

3   For the patties, stir in the onion, garlic and the beetroot grated into the millet. Let cool down. Then stir the flour into the millet mixture. Season with salt and pepper. Shape the mixture into 12 flat thalers.

4   Chop the walnut kernels, toast in a large non-stick pan, remove. Heat 1 tablespoon of oil in the pan, fry the patties for 3–4 minutes on each side.

5   For the vinaigrette, stir together vinegar, 2 teaspoons of mustard, salt and pepper. Stir in 2 tablespoons of oil. Spread the lamb's lettuce, radish and walnuts on four plates. Drizzle with the vinaigrette. Place the patties on top and serve the quark dip.

Nutritional info

1 portion approx:

400 kcal17 g protein15 g fat43 g of carbohydrates

Zucchini dumplings in a tomato and coconut sauce

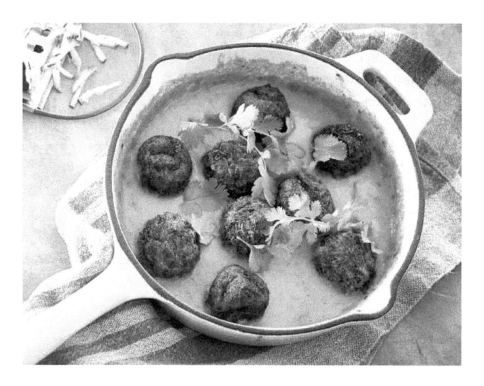

Ingredients For 4 people

- 250 g floury potatoes
- 500 g zucchini
- salt
- Chilli flakes
- pepper
- sugar
- Spring onions
- 1 federal government coriander
- 300 g tomatoes
- 1 piece (s) (approx. 20 g each) ginger
- 1 tbsp Sunflower oil
- 100 ml Sunflower oil
- Bay leaf
- 1 tbsp Garam Masala (Indian spice mix)
- 250 ml unsweetened coconut milk
- 2 tbsp Lime juice
- 2 tbsp Flour
- something Flour

preparation

50 minutes

1. For the köfte, cook the potatoes in boiling water for about 20 minutes. Clean, wash and coarsely grate the zucchini. Knead in 1 teaspoon of salt and let it steep for about 20 minutes. Clean and wash the spring onions and cut into fine rings. Wash the coriander, shake dry and chop finely. Drain the potatoes, rinse in cold water, peel.

2. For the sauce, wash and dice tomatoes. Peel the ginger and grate finely. Heat 1 tablespoon of oil in a saucepan. Sauté tomatoes, ginger and bay leaves in it for about 3 minutes. Take out the bay leaves. Add garam masala and coconut milk and puree finely. Season to taste with chilli flakes, lime juice, salt, pepper and sugar.

3. Coarsely grate the potatoes and squeeze out the zucchini in portions. Mix both with chopped coriander, spring onions and 5 tbsp flour. Season the mixture with pepper and possibly salt and form approx. 16 balls out of it with floured hands.

4. Heat approx. 100 ml of oil in a large pan. Fry the zucchini pots all around for about 5 minutes. Remove from the pan and drain briefly on kitchen paper, then add the kofte to the sauce.

Nutritional info

1 portion approx:

300 kcal7 g protein14 g fat34 g of carbohydrates

Fish gratin with spinach

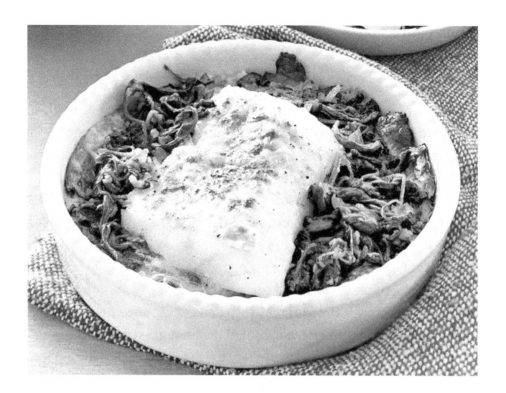

Ingredients For 4 people

- 1 kg young spinach leaves
- 1 Onion, 1 clove of garlic
- 1 tbsp Oil, salt, pepper, nutmeg
- 150 ml Milk, 3 eggs (size M)
- 650 g Fish fillet (e.g. saithe)
- 1 tbsp Lemon juice
- 50 g Emmentaler (piece)

preparation

60 minutes

1 Clean, wash and drain the spinach. Peel onion and garlic and chop finely. Heat the oil in the pan. Sauté the onion and garlic in it. Add the spinach, cover and collapse. Season with salt, pepper and nutmeg.

2 Preheat the oven (electric stove: 200 ° C / convection: 175 ° C / gas: see manufacturer). Whisk the milk and eggs together. Season with salt and pepper. Rinse the fish, pat dry, cut into 4 pieces. Drizzle with lemon, lightly salt.

3   Divide the spinach into four ovenproof dishes (or one large dish). Place 1 fillet on each. Baste with egg milk. Rub cheese over it. Bake in the oven for about 20 minutes.

Nutritional info

1 person approx:

270 kcal41 g protein10 g fat3 g of carbohydrates

Baked schnitzel pan

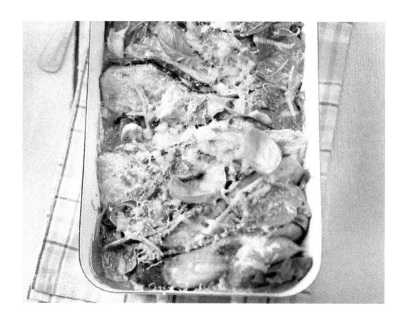

Ingredients For 4 people

- 1 large eggplant (approx. 400 g)
- salt
- 4th tomatoes
- 200 g Baby spinach
- Garlic cloves
- 1 small onion
- 1 tbsp butter
- pepper
- grated nutmeg
- 6th Pork schnitzel (approx. 125 g each)
- 5 1/2 tbsp oil
- 1 can (s) (425 ml) sieved tomatos
- 150 ml Vegetable broth
- 1 tbsp dark balsamic vinegar
- stem (s) basil
- sugar
- 50 g Parmesan cheese
- fat

preparation

45 minutes

1   Clean the aubergine and cut into 8–10 slices. Sprinkle the slices with salt on both sides and place on kitchen paper. Wash, clean and halve tomatoes. Clean and wash the spinach. Peel the garlic and onion and finely dice up to 1/2 clove. Melt 1 tbsp butter in a saucepan. Sauté the onion and half of the garlic in it. Add the spinach and 3–4 tablespoons of water and cook for 2–3 minutes, turning. Season with salt, pepper and nutmeg. If necessary, pound the meat flat and season with salt and pepper. Rub the pan with 1/2 clove of garlic. Heat 3 tablespoons of oil in portions. Sear the aubergine slices in approx. 3 portions on both sides, remove. Put 2 tablespoons of oil in the pan. Fry the schnitzel in 2 portions on both sides, remove. Put the rest of the garlic and 1/2 teaspoon of oil in the pan and sauté briefly.

2   Add the strained tomatoes, stock and vinegar and simmer for about 4 minutes. In the meantime, wash the basil, pat dry and cut into fine strips, except for something to garnish. Season the tomato sauce with salt, pepper and sugar. Stir in the basil. Coat the baking dish with fat. Alternately add aubergine slices, halved tomatoes, schnitzel and spinach and baste with tomato sauce. Bake in a preheated oven (electric stove: 200 ° C / fan: 175 ° C / gas: level 3) for 12–15 minutes.

3   Finely grate the parmesan and sprinkle over it approx. 5 minutes before the end of the cooking time Coat the baking dish with fat. Alternately add aubergine slices, halved tomatoes, schnitzel and spinach and baste with tomato sauce. Bake in a preheated oven (electric stove: 200 ° C / fan: 175 ° C / gas: level 3) for 12–15 minutes. Finely grate the parmesan and sprinkle over it approx. 5 minutes before the end of the cooking time Coat the baking dish with fat. Alternately add aubergine slices, halved tomatoes, schnitzel and spinach and baste with tomato sauce. Bake in a preheated oven (electric stove: 200 ° C / fan: 175 ° C / gas: level 3) for 12–15 minutes. Finely grate the parmesan and sprinkle over it approx. 5 minutes before the end of the cooking time

Nutritional info

1 person approx:

310 kcal1300 kJ34 g protein15 g fat8 g of carbohydrates

Eggplant and tomato casserole with beef mince

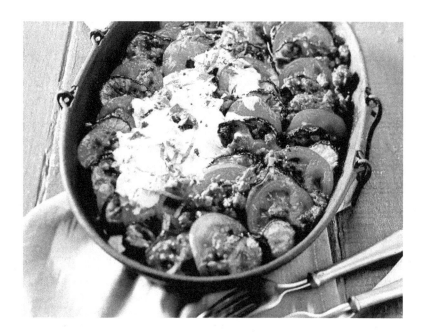

Ingredients For 4 people

- 2 large eggplant
- salt
- Cayenne pepper
- coriander
- pepper
- 4 tbsp olive oil
- Onions
- 250 g Beefsteakhack
- 3 tbsp Tomato paste
- 4th tomatoes
- 1 clove of garlic
- stem / s mint
- 300 g Whole milk yogurt

preparation

50 minutes (+ 60 minutes waiting time)

1   Clean and wash the aubergines, cut into approx. 1 cm thick slices. Sprinkle a baking
    sheet with 1 teaspoon of salt. Spread the slices on top, sprinkle with about 1 teaspoon
    of salt. Let the aubergines steep for about 1 hour.

2   Pat the eggplants dry. Pat the tray dry, brush with 1 tbsp oil. Spread the aubergines on
    top and brush with 2 tablespoons of oil. Fry the aubergine slices under the hot grill for

about 15 minutes, turning once.

3   For the minced sauce, peel and finely dice the onions. Heat 1 tablespoon of oil in a pan. Fry the mince in it finely, fry the onions briefly. Stir in tomato paste and 150 ml water, bring to the boil. Season with salt, cayenne pepper and 1 teaspoon coriander.

4   Preheat the oven (electric stove: 200 ° C / convection: 180 ° C / gas: see manufacturer). Wash, clean and slice tomatoes. Put half of the sauce in a baking dish. Layer the eggplants and tomatoes. Season with salt and pepper. Spread the rest of the sauce over it. Close the tin with aluminum foil and bake in the hot oven for about 15 minutes.

5   Peel and chop the garlic. Wash the mint, shake dry, pluck off the leaves and cut into strips. Mix both with yogurt. Season with salt and pepper. Spread some yoghurt on the casserole, serve the rest.

Nutritional info

1 portion approx:

300 kcal22 g protein16 g fat15 g of carbohydrates

Thai vegetable stir-fry with sesame meatballs

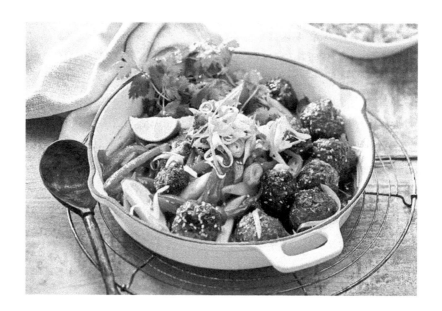

Ingredients For 4 people

- 500 g broccoli
- 1 red pepper
- 1/2 bunch Spring onions
- 1 onion
- Garlic cloves
- 1 piece (s) (approx. 30 g each) ginger
- 600 g Beefsteakhack (tartare)
- 3 tbsp lowfat quark
- salt
- pepper
- 2 tbsp oil
- 2 Organic limes
- 1/2 mango
- 3 tbsp Soy sauce
- 1 tbsp sesame

some stem / s Coriander for garnish

preparation

35 minutes

1   Clean and wash broccoli and cut into small florets. Clean and wash the peppers and cut into strips. Clean and wash the spring onions and cut into fine rings.

2   Preheat the oven (electric stove: 150 ° C / convection: 130 ° C / gas: see manufacturer). Peel onion and garlic and chop finely. Peel the ginger and grate finely. Knead the mince, quark, onion, garlic and ginger well. Season with about 1 teaspoon of salt and 1⁄2 teaspoon of pepper. Shape the mixture into about 16 balls. Heat the oil in a large pan (with a lid). Fry the meatballs all around for about 4 minutes, remove them and spread them on a baking sheet. Finish cooking in the hot oven for approx. 10 minutes.

3   Cover the broccoli and bell peppers in the hot frying fat for 4–5 minutes. Turn in between. Wash limes with hot water, dry. Halve and squeeze 1 lime, cut 1 into wedges. Peel the mango, cut the flesh off the stone and into wedges. Deglaze the vegetables with the soy sauce and lime juice. Fold in mango slices, heat briefly. Season with pepper.

4   Arrange the vegetables and meatballs and sprinkle with spring onions and sesame seeds. Garnish with lime wedges and coriander.

Nutritional info

1 portion approx:

360 kcal39 g protein16 g fat13 g of carbohydrates

Carrot and fish ragout with chili

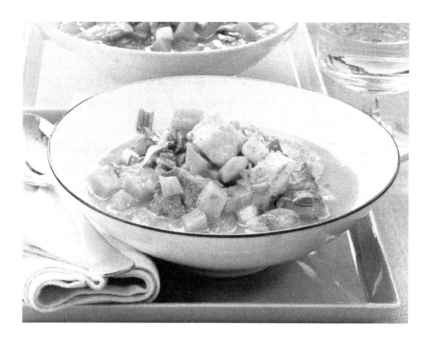

Ingredients For 4 people

- 1 onion
- Chilli pepper
- 400 g Carrots
- 1 federal government Spring onions
- 600 g Pollack fillet
- 2 tbsp oil
- salt
- pepper
- Curry powder
- 1 tsp Vegetable broth (instant)
- 2 tsp food starch

preparation

30 minutes

1. Peel and dice the onion. Cut the chilli open, remove the seeds, wash and chop. Peel or clean the carrots and spring onions, wash and cut into small pieces.
2. Rinse the fish, pat dry, chop roughly. Fry in hot oil, season with salt and pepper, remove. Sauté the prepared ingredients and 2 teaspoons of curry in the frying fat. Add 400 ml of water and stock, bring to the boil and simmer for about 10 minutes.
3. Mix starch with 2 tablespoons of water, bind the curry with it. Heat the fish in it. In addition: rice.

Nutritional info

1 person approx:

220 kcal29 g protein6 g fat11 g of carbohydrates

Lentil salad with fried apples

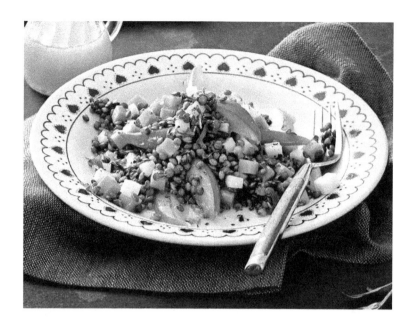

Ingredients For 4 people

- 200 g green puy lentils
- 2 big carrots
- Parsley roots or
- 1/2 celery root
- Salt pepper
- 4 tbsp Apple Cider Vinegar
- 1 tbsp Liquid honey
- 1 tbsp oil
- 1/2 bunch flat leaf parsley
- 3 Apples (e.g. Elstar)
- 1 tbsp butter

preparation

35 minutes

1 Rinse the lentils with cold water, then cook in boiling water for about 20 minutes. Peel and wash the carrots and parsley roots and cut into small cubes. Add to the lentils about 5 minutes before the end of the cooking time, season with salt and continue cooking.
2 Drain, rinse with cold water and drain well.
3 Mix the vinegar, honey, salt and pepper together. Beat the oil on it. Wash the parsley and shake dry, pluck the leaves from the stems and cut into fine strips. Mix the vinaigrette and parsley with the lentil vegetables.

4   Wash the apples, quarter them and remove the core. Cut apple quarters into wedges. Heat the butter in a pan and fry the apples until golden.

Nutritional info

1 person approx:

310 kcal15 g protein6 g fat46 g of carbohydrates

Asian mushroom omelette

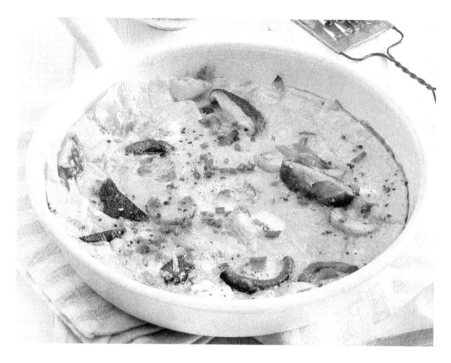

Ingredients For 4 people

- 4th Spring onions
- red chilli pepper
- 20 g Ginger tuber
- 200 g Shiitake mushrooms
- 200 g Mushrooms
- 4 tsp sesame oil
- salt
- pepper
- 12th Eggs (size M)
- 8th Stalks of chives
- coarse pepper

preparation

30 minutes

1   Clean and wash the spring onions and cut into thin rings. Wash the chilli and cut into fine rings. Ginger peel and finely chop. Clean the mushrooms and cut in half.

2   Heat 1 teaspoon of oil in each of two pans (21 cm Ø), fry 1/4 of the ingredients in each, season with salt and pepper. In the meantime, whisk the eggs, season with salt and pepper and add 1/4 of the egg mixture to both pans and cover and let stand for 10-15 minutes over a low heat.

3   Place the omelets on a baking sheet and keep them warm in the oven at 50 ° C.
4   Bake the remaining ingredients for 2 more omelets. Wash the chives, shake dry and cut into fine rolls. Sprinkle the omelets with coarse pepper and chives.

Nutritional info

1 person approx:

370 kcal1550 kJ26 g protein26 g fat10 g of carbohydrates

(Vietnamese noodle soup with beef)

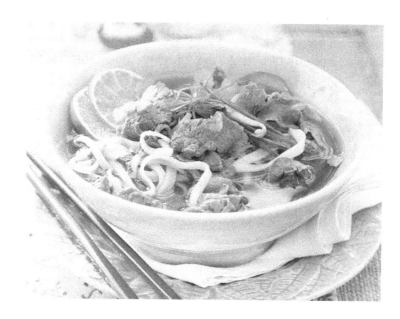

Ingredients For 4 people

- 500 g Soupmeat
- salt
- 50 g fresh ginger
- 2 Star anise
- 1 onion
- 1 federal government Soup greens
- 250 g Flat rice noodles
- 300 g Beef fillet
- 50 g Mung Bean Sprouts
- 2 Spring onions
- 1/2 Pot of coriander
- 4 stem (s) peppermint
- lime
- 4 tbsp Soy sauce

pepper

preparation

135 minutes

1   Wash the meat of the soup and cook in approx. 2 liters of boiling, lightly salted water for approx. 2 hours. Wash the ginger and cut into thin slices. Season the broth with star anise and ginger. Clean the onion, cut in half across the flower and root and fry in a pan

without fat over medium heat for about 10 minutes.

2   Clean the soup greens, if necessary peel, wash and cut into pieces. Add the soup vegetables and onions to the meat about 1 1/2 hours before the end of the cooking time. Prepare the pasta in boiling salted water according to the instructions on the packet.

3   Wash the beef fillet, pat dry and cut into very thin slices. Wash the bean sprouts. Clean and wash the spring onions and cut into very thin rings. Wash the herbs, shake dry and, except for something to garnish, pluck leaves from the stems and chop.

4   Pour the stock through a sieve, use the soup meat otherwise. Wash the lime in hot water, rub dry, cut the fruit in half. Squeeze half, cut the other half into slices. Season the broth with soy sauce, lime juice and pepper to taste, bring to the boil.

5   Drain the pasta in a colander, drain. Arrange the pasta, vegetables, herbs and meat in soup bowls and pour the hot broth over them. Garnish with the lime and the rest of the coriander.

Nutritional info

1 person approx:

360 kcal1510 kJ23 g protein5 g of fat56 g of carbohydrates

Cauliflower and lentil curry

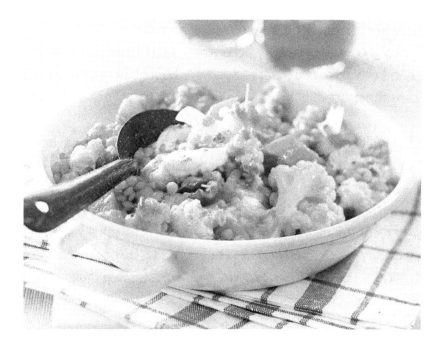

Ingredients For 4 people

- 1 Cauliflower (approx. 1 kg)
- 2 big carrots
- 50-75 g dried pitted dates or raisins
- 2 tbsp oil
- salt and pepper
- 1-2 tsp curry
- 200 g Red lenses
- 2 stem (s) Coriander or parsley
- 200 g Cream yogurt (e.g. Greek)
- 1 tsp food starch

preparation

30 minutes

1 Clean and wash the cauliflower and cut into small florets. Peel and wash the carrots, halve lengthways and cut into pieces. Cut the dates into slices.

2 Heat the oil in a large, tall pan (with a lid). Fry the cauliflower and carrots in it. Season with salt and pepper. Add the lentils and dates and sauté briefly. Dust with curry and sweat.

3 Pour in 1 / 2–3 / 4 l of water, bring to the boil and simmer covered for approx. 10 minutes. Stirring occasionally.

4 Wash the coriander, shake dry and pluck the leaves off. Mix approx. 3/4 yoghurt and starch until smooth. Stir under the lentils and briefly (!) Bring to the boil while stirring. Season to taste with salt, pepper and possibly a little curry.

5 Serve the cauliflower curry with the rest of the yogurt and sprinkle with coriander leaves. Indian flatbread tastes good with it.

Drink tip: cool iced tea or mango lassi.

Nutritional info

1 person approx:

380 kcal19 g protein11 g fat48 g of carbohydrates

Carrot and Quinoa Soup

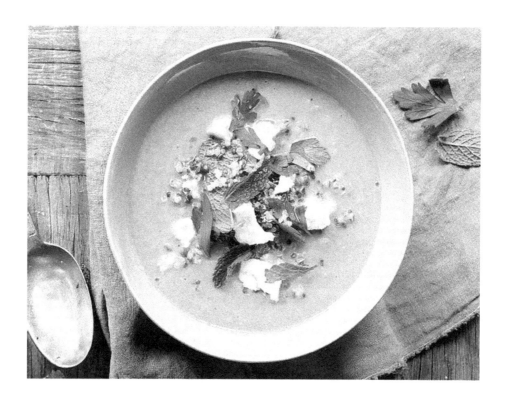

Ingredients For 4 people

- 1.2 kg Carrots
- Organic lemons
- 100 g Quinoa
- 10 stem / s Herbs (e.g. parsley and mint)
- 300 g Double cream cheese
- 1 onion
- 2 Garlic cloves
- Salt, ground cumin, sweet paprika, pepper
- 2 tbsp olive oil
- 2 tbsp Vegetable broth (instant)

preparation

45 minutes

1   Peel, wash and finely dice the carrots. Peel the onion and garlic, dice both finely. Wash the lemons, dry them, rub the peel. Squeeze fruits. Rinse the quinoa with hot water and cook in 1⁄4 l salted water for about 15 minutes.

2   In the meantime, sauté the carrots, onions and garlic in the hot oil. Dust with 1 teaspoon of cumin and 1 teaspoon of paprika, sauté. Add 1.4 liters of water and stock, bring to the

boil. Simmer for about 10 minutes.

3   Wash and pluck herbs. Add lemon zest, juice and half of the cheese to the soup, puree. Season with salt and pepper. Serve with quinoa, the rest of the cheese and herbs. In addition: flat bread.

Nutritional info

1 portion approx:

280 kcal6 g protein17 g fat24 g of carbohydrates

Sweet potato tarte flambée with harissa cream

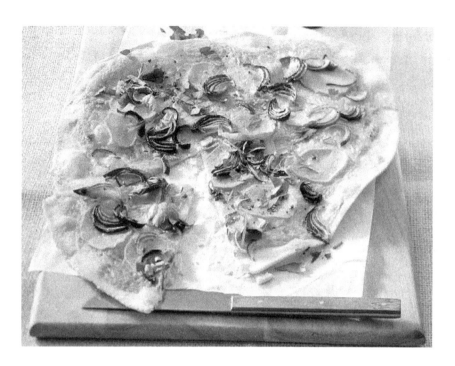

Ingredients For 4 people

- 1 pack (260 g) fresh tarte flambée batter (approx. 40 x 24 cm; refrigerated shelf)
- 300 g sour cream
- 2 tbsp Harissa (Arabic spice paste; tube)
- salt
- 2 Red onions
- 1–2 (approx. 300 g) Sweet potatoes
- 3–4 stem (s) flat leaf parsley

preparation

25 minutes

1 Take the dough out of the refrigerator and let it rest at room temperature for about 10 minutes. Preheat the oven (electric stove: 250 ° C / convection: 225 ° C / gas: see manufacturer).

2 For the cream, mix together the sour cream and harissa. Season to taste with salt. Peel the onions and cut into strips. Peel and wash sweet potatoes and slice or cut them into very thin slices.

3 Unroll the dough and place on a baking sheet with the baking paper. Brush with harissa cream and top with sweet potatoes and onions.

4 Bake in the hot oven for 10–12 minutes. In the meantime, wash the parsley, shake dry, pluck the leaves from the stalks and roughly chop. Sprinkle the tarte flambée with

parsley.

Nutritional info

1 person approx:

360 kcal

Stuffed ox heart tomatoes with quinoa and cottage cheese

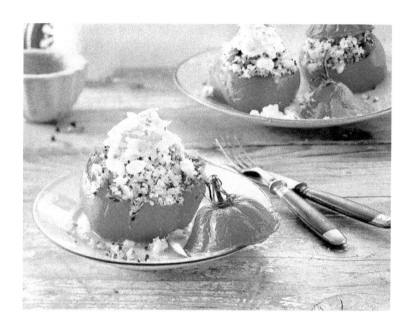

Ingredients For 4 people

- 200 g Quinoa
- salt
- 4th Oxheart tomatoes (approx. 300 g each)
- 1/2 bunch Spring onions
- 250 g cottage cheese
- pepper

preparation

30 minutes

1   Put the quinoa in a fine sieve, rinse thoroughly and cook in 600 ml salted water according to the instructions on the packet. In the meantime, wash the tomatoes, cut off a lid on the stem side and hollow out the tomatoes.

2   Wash and clean the spring onions and cut into fine rings. Drain the quinoa and rinse with cold water. Mix the quinoa, about half of the spring onions and about half of the cottage cheese, season with salt and pepper.

3   Fill the tomatoes with the quinoa mixture and place the lids on a baking sheet. Bake in a preheated oven (electric stove: 175 ° C / convection: 150 ° C / gas: see manufacturer) for about 12 minutes. Take the tomatoes out of the oven, spread the remaining cottage cheese and spring onion rings on top and serve.

Nutritional info

1 person approx:

270 kcal1130 kJ18 g protein4 g of fat40 g of carbohydrates

Stuffed zucchini with ricotta and ham

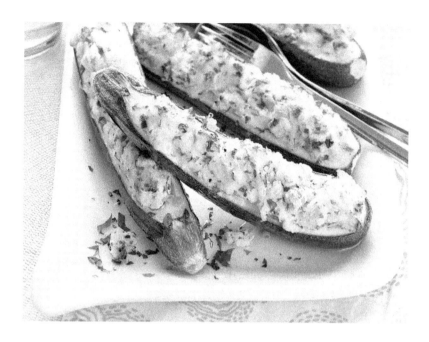

Ingredients For 4 people

- discs White bread from the previous day
- 150 ml milk
- 4th small zucchini (approx. 150 g each)
- handle (s) basil
- 1/2 bunch parsley
- 2 Garlic cloves
- 2 discs cooked ham (approx. 30 g each)
- 125 g Ricotta cheese
- 1 Egg (size M)
- 3 tbsp oil

salt

pepper

fat

preparation

45 minutes

1 Soak the bread in milk for about 15 minutes. Clean and wash the zucchini, cut off the upper third lengthways. Carefully hollow out the zucchini. Chop the pulp. Wash the herbs, shake dry, pluck the leaves off and cut into small pieces. Peel garlic and chop

finely. Cut ham into strips.

2 Lightly squeeze out the bread, mix with the ricotta, egg, 2 tablespoons of oil, 3/4 of the herbs, garlic, zucchini pulp and strips of ham, season with salt and pepper.

3 Fill the hollowed-out zucchini with the mixture, place in a greased baking dish. Drizzle with 1 tablespoon of oil and bake in the preheated oven (electric stove: 175 ° C / fan: 150 ° C / gas: level 2) for about 25 minutes. Remove the zucchini, arrange and sprinkle with the remaining herbs.

Nutritional info

1 person approx:

230 kcal960 kJ12 g protein16 g fat12 g of carbohydrates

Stir-fried fillet with sesame

vegetables

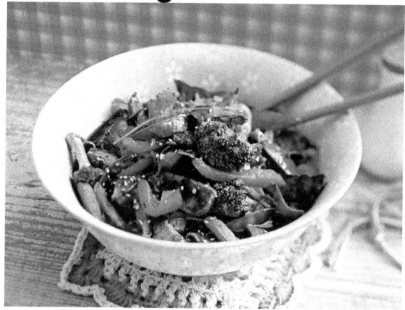

Ingredients For 4 people

- 500 g broccoli
- 1 red pepper
- 200 g sugar snap
- red chilli pepper
- 600 g pork tenderloin
- 2 tbsp sesame
- 4 tbsp oil
- 100 ml Soy sauce
- 1-2 tbsp Liquid honey
- 1 tsp Asian spice
- 1 tsp food starch
- 4–5 stem (s) coriander

preparation

30 minutes

1   Trim and wash broccoli and cut into florets. Clean and wash the peppers and cut into strips. Wash and clean the sugar snap peas and cut in half at an angle. Clean the chilli, cut lengthways, core, wash and cut into small pieces.
2   Pat the meat dry and cut into thin strips.

3   Roast the sesame seeds in a wok or a large pan without fat, remove. Heat the oil in the wok. Fry the meat in 2 portions, turning for about 3 minutes, remove. Fry the broccoli and paprika in the hot frying fat, stirring constantly, for 3–4 minutes.
4   Fry the sugar snap peas briefly.
5   Add the soy sauce, 100 ml water, honey and Asian spices, bring to the boil. Mix the starch and 1 tbsp water until smooth. Tie the sauce with it. Reheat the meat in it. Wash the coriander, shake dry and pluck the leaves.
6   Scatter coriander and sesame seeds on top. In addition: rice.

Nutritional info

1 person approx:

360 kcal39 g protein11 g fat23 g of carbohydrates

Fixed kale minestrone

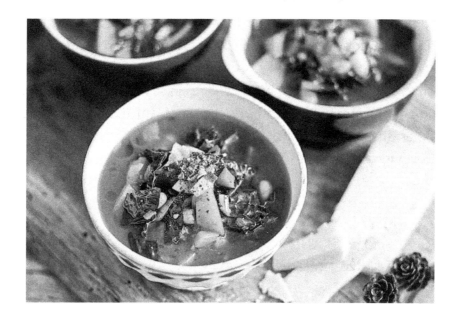

Ingredients For 4 people

- 2 Onions
- 3 Garlic cloves
- 4th Carrots
- 2 Parsnips
- 5 tbsp olive oil
- 1 pack (500 ml each) sieved tomatos
- 1 tbsp Vegetable broth (instant)
- 1 can (s) (425 ml each) White beans
- zucchini
- 300 g cleaned kale
- Salt pepper

preparation

25 minutes

1. Peel and chop the onions and garlic. Peel, wash and chop the carrots and parsnips.
2. Braise the prepared ingredients in the hot oil. Add the strained tomatoes, 1 1/2 l water and stock and bring to the boil. Cover and simmer for 10–12 minutes.
3. In the meantime, rinse and drain the beans. Clean, wash and dice the zucchini. Wash the cabbage well and cut into strips. Add the beans, zucchini and cabbage about 5 minutes

before the end of the cooking time. Season to taste with salt and pepper.

Nutritional info

1 portion approx:

280 kcal13 g protein12 g fat28 g of carbohydrates

Balsamic sprouts with turkey strips

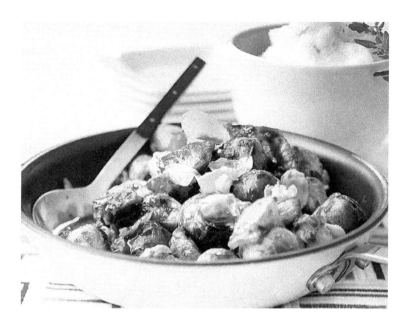

Ingredients For 2 people

- 400 g Brussels sprouts
- Salt, pepper, nutmeg
- 500 g Potatoes
- 1 small onion
- 250 g Turkey schnitzel
- 1 tbsp oil
- 1/2 tsp Brown sugar
- 2 tbsp Balsamic vinegar
- 100 ml milk

preparation

40 minutes

1   Clean and wash the Brussels sprouts, cover and cook in a little salted water for about 15 minutes. Peel, wash and roughly dice the potatoes and cook covered in boiling salted water for about 20 minutes.
2   In the meantime, peel and finely dice the onion. Rinse the meat, pat dry and cut into strips. Heat oil in a pan. Fry the meat in it over a high heat for 3-4 minutes. Season with salt and pepper. Remove.
3   Drain the Brussels sprouts. Fry the onion and Brussels sprouts in the frying oil for about 3 minutes. Sprinkle with sugar and fry for 2-3 minutes. Add vinegar, 1⁄8 l water and meat and simmer for 5 minutes. Season everything with salt and pepper.

4   Drain the potatoes. Pour in milk and mash everything. Season with salt and nutmeg. Serve everything.

Nutritional info

1 person approx:

400 kcal37 g protein9 g fat40 g of carbohydrates

Bell pepper couscous as a turbo salad

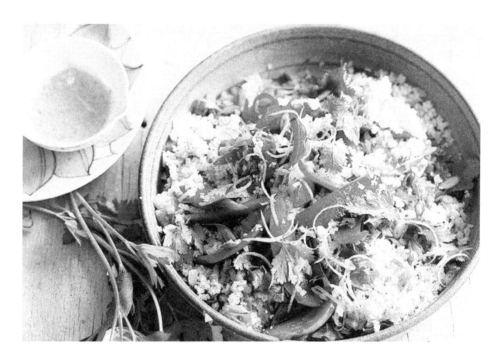

Ingredients For 4 people

- 200 g couscous
- Salt pepper
- 2 red peppers
- 2 Spring onions
- 1/2 bunch Coriander and parsley
- 1 Organic lemon
- 1 tbsp Maple syrup
- 6 tbsp olive oil

preparation

25 minutes

1. Mix the couscous with 1⁄4 teaspoon of salt, pour 1⁄4 l of boiling water over it and cover it for approx. 5 minutes.
2. Clean and wash the peppers and cut into strips. Clean and wash the spring onions and cut into fine rings. Wash the herbs, shake dry, pluck the leaves off and cut roughly. Fluff the couscous with a fork, mix in the prepared ingredients.
3. Wash the lemon with hot water, dry it and peel off some of the peel in thin strips. Squeeze the lemon. Mix together the juice, salt, pepper and maple syrup, fold in the oil. Mix the lemon vinaigrette with the salad and sprinkle with lemon zest.

Nutritional info

1 portion approx:

260 kcal4 g protein17 g fat21 g of carbohydrates

Fruity asparagus salad with quinoa

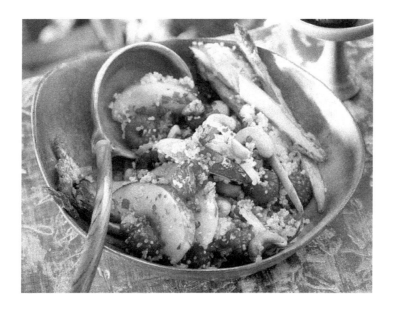

Ingredients For 4 people

- 200 g white quinoa
- Salt pepper
- 4 tbsp Lime juice
- 4 tbsp oil
- 500 g green asparagus
- 2 tbsp Cashew nuts
- 4 Nectarines
- 150 g Raspberries
- 2 Spring onions
- 1 federal government flat leaf parsley

preparation

45 minutes

1   Rinse and drain quinoa. Bring 400 ml water and 1⁄2 teaspoon salt to the boil. Stir in the quinoa and simmer over low heat for about 15 minutes until the water is soaked up. Stirring occasionally. Take it from the stove and let it cool off.

2   Mix the lime juice, salt and pepper together. Beat in 2 tbsp oil. Mix the vinaigrette and quinoa.

3   Wash the asparagus, cut off the woody ends. Halve the sticks lengthways and crossways. Roast cashew nuts in a pan without fat. Remove. Heat 2 tablespoons of oil in the pan, fry the asparagus in it for about 4 minutes.

4   Season with salt and pepper.

5   Wash the nectarines, cut in half, stone and cut into wedges. Sort out raspberries, rinse if necessary. Clean and wash the spring onions and cut into rings. Wash parsley, shake dry and finely chop.
6   Mix the quinoa, asparagus and the other prepared ingredients.

Nutritional info

1 person approx:

400 kcal12 g protein17 g fat48 g of carbohydrates

Turbo glass noodle salad with mince

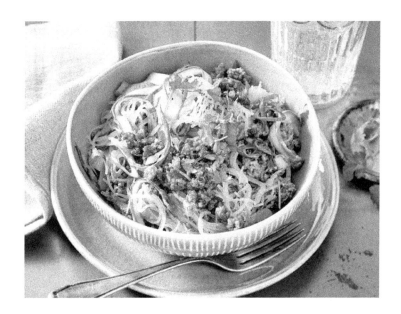

Ingredients For 4 people

- 200 g Glass noodles
- 300 g green asparagus
- 5 tbsp oil
- salt
- pepper
- Chilli flakes
- 400 g mixed hack
- 1 pc. (approx. 20 g) ginger
- 2 Spring onions
- Juice of 1 lime
- 4 tbsp Fish sauce
- 1/2 tsp honey
- 1/2 bunch coriander

preparation

30 minutes

1 Pour boiling water over glass noodles, leave to soak for about 10 minutes. Wash the asparagus, cut off the woody ends. Cut the asparagus lengthways into strips with the peeler. Fry in 2 tablespoons of hot oil for about 4 minutes, season with salt, remove.

2 Fry the mince in the frying fat until crumbly. Peel and chop the ginger. Wash and clean the spring onions and cut into rings. Fry both briefly. Season with salt and pepper.

3   Mix together the lime juice, fish sauce, honey, chilli and 3 tablespoons of oil. Mix the drained pasta, asparagus, mince and sauce. Wash, chop and sprinkle the coriander.

Nutritional info

1 portion approx:

510 kcal23 g protein33 g fat26 g of carbohydrates

Asian carrot and pepper soup

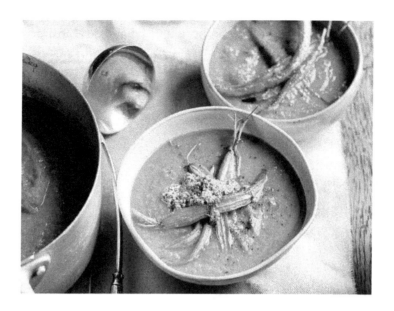

Ingredients For 4 people

- 1 kg Carrots
- 2 Onions
- 1 red pepper
- 2 tbsp oil
- 1 tsp Red curry paste
- 2 tbsp Brown sugar
- 2-3 tbsp Lemon juice
- 4 tsp Vegetable broth (instant)
- 4-6 tbsp light soy sauce

preparation

30 minutes

1. Peel and wash the carrots. Peel the onions. Clean and wash the peppers. Cut everything into 1–2 cm pieces.
2. Heat oil in a pot. Lightly fry the carrots, bell peppers and onions for about 2 minutes while stirring. Stir in curry paste. Sprinkle with sugar and deglaze with 2 tablespoons of lemon juice. Add about 3⁄4 l of hot water. Stir in the broth. Cover and cook for 15–20 minutes.
3. Finely puree the carrots with a hand blender, adding approx. 300 ml of hot water to the desired consistency. Briefly bring the soup to the boil. Season with soy sauce and lemon

juice. Serve with Thai vials and coriander pesto as desired.

Nutritional info

1 portion approx:

140 kcal3 g protein6 g fat16 g of carbohydrates

Coconut Lime Fish

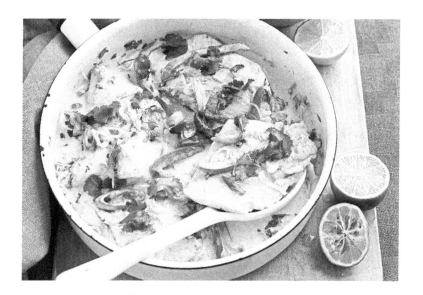

Ingredients For 4 people

- 1 clove of garlic
- 1 piece (approx. 2 cm) ginger
- 1 big red chili pepper
- 1 red pepper
- Spring onions
- 1 Organic lime
- 4 pieces Cod fillet (approx. 150 g each)
- 3 tbsp oil
- Salt, pepper, sugar
- 1 can (s) (400 ml each) unsweetened coconut milk
- 5 stems coriander

preparation

35 minutes

1 Peel and finely chop the garlic and ginger. Clean the chilli peppers, cut lengthways, core, wash and finely chop. Clean and wash the peppers and cut into thin strips. Clean and wash the spring onions and cut into rings. Wash the lime with hot, dry it and rub the peel. Halve and squeeze the lime.

2 Rinse the fish and pat dry well. Heat 2 tablespoons of oil in a large pan. Fry the fish in it over medium heat for about 2 minutes on each side. Season with salt and remove.

3   Heat 1 tablespoon of oil in the frying fat. Sauté the garlic, ginger, chilli and paprika in it
    for 2-3 minutes. Deglaze with coconut milk and 1⁄8 l water, season with salt and pepper.
    Bring to a boil. Add the fish and cover everything and simmer over a low heat for about
    5 minutes.
4   Wash the coriander, shake dry, pull off the leaves. Stir the spring onions, lime juice and
    zest into the coconut sauce. Season with salt, pepper and sugar. Sprinkle with the
    coriander leaves.

Nutritional info

1 portion approx:

440 kcal33 g protein28 g fat10 g of carbohydrates

omelette with salmon and fennel salad

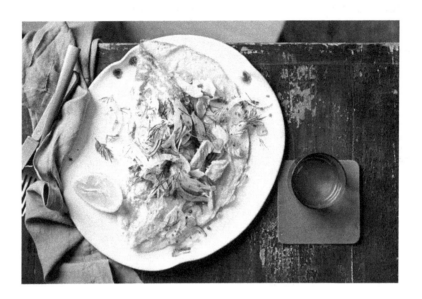

Ingredients For 2 people

- 1/2 fennel
- 1 small red onion
- 2 stems dill
- stalks chives
- 1/2 Organic lemon
- Salt pepper
- 1 tbsp olive oil
- 2 tsp olive oil
- 5 Eggs (size M)
- 100 g Creme fraiche Cheese
- 2 tsp butter
- 75 g Stremel salmon

preparation

25 minutes

1   Clean the fennel (put the greens aside), wash and slice or cut into very fine slices. Peel the onion and cut into fine strips. Wash the dill, fennel greens and chives, shake dry and

roughly chop or cut into rolls. Mix everything with lemon juice, salt, pepper and 1 tablespoon of oil.

2   Whisk eggs, crème fraîche and lemon zest together. Season with 1⁄2 teaspoon salt and 1⁄4 teaspoon pepper. Heat 1 teaspoon each of oil and butter in a pan. Pour in half of the egg mixture and let it set briefly over low to medium heat. Turn and finish baking. Keep warm. Bake a second omelette using the rest of the oil, butter and egg mixture. Serve with the shredded salmon and fennel salad.

Nutritional info

1 portion approx:

560 kcal28 g protein44 g fat8 g of carbohydrates

Spicy Chicken Wrap

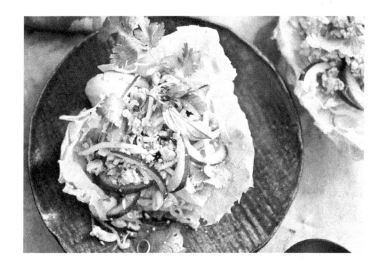

Ingredients For 2 people

- 400 g Chicken fillet
- 2 tbsp olive oil
- Salt pepper
- Mini cucumber
- Red onion
- 30 g Mung bean sprouts
- red chilli pepper
- clove of garlic
- 2 tbsp light soy sauce
- 1 tbsp Agave syrup
- 1/2 lime
- 3 tbsp unsalted peanuts
- 4th large leaves of iceberg lettuce
- 2 stems Coriander and Thai basil

preparation

30 minutes

1   Wash the chicken, pat dry and dice, then chop very finely. Heat oil in a large pan. Fry the meat in it for 3-4 minutes, turning. Season with salt and pepper, remove.
2   Wash the cucumber, cut in half lengthways, core and cut into thin slices. Peel the onion and cut into fine strips. Sort out the sprouts, wash them and let them drain.
3   For the dressing, clean and wash the chilli and finely chop the kernels. Peel garlic and chop finely. Mix both with soy sauce, 1 tbsp water, agave syrup and lime juice.
4   Mix the prepared ingredients and dressing. Chop nuts. Wash the lettuce leaves, shake well dry and fill with the chicken salad. Sprinkle with the peanuts. Serve with coriander and Thai basil if you like.

Nutritional info

1 portion approx:

460 kcal47 g protein24 g fat10 g of carbohydrates

Bargain salad with crispy feta

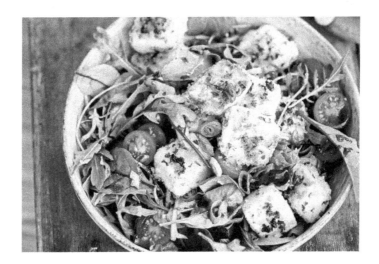

Ingredients For 2 people

- 5 stems oregano
- 1 clove of garlic
- 2 packs (200 g each) Feta
- 8 tbsp olive oil
- 4 tbsp Panko (Japanese breadcrumbs; alternatively, breadcrumbs)
- 250 g Cherry tomatoes
- 100 g Baby salad mix
- 2 Spring onions
- 4 tbsp Balsamic vinegar
- Salt, pepper, sugar
- Parchment paper

preparation

25 minutes

1   Preheat for the feta oven (electric stove: 240 ° C / convection: 220 ° C / gas: see
    manufacturer). Line a tray with baking paper. Wash the oregano, shake dry, remove the
    leaves. Peel the garlic. Finely chop both. Cut the feta into approx. 2 cm cubes. Mix
    carefully with oregano, garlic, 5 tablespoons oil and panko. Spread on the baking sheet

and bake in the hot oven for about 10 minutes.

2   Wash and halve tomatoes for the salad. Sort out the salad mix, wash, spin dry. Clean and wash the spring onions and cut into fine rings. Mix the vinegar, salt, pepper and sugar together. Beat in 3 tablespoons of oil. Mix the lettuce, tomatoes, spring onions and vinaigrette together. Take the cheese out of the oven and place on the salad.

Nutritional info

1 portion approx:

530 kcal18 g protein45 g fat9 g of carbohydrates

Fat burner bowl with mince and silken tofu

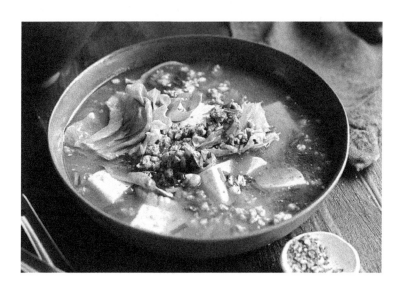

Ingredients For 4 people

- 8 tbsp Rice wine (alternatively sherry)
- 8 tbsp Soy sauce
- 400 g Ground beef
- 1 piece (approx. 30 g each) ginger
- 2 Garlic cloves
- 1 tbsp oil
- 1 tsp coarsely ground Szechuan pepper
- 1 tbsp Chilli Bean Sauce (Asian Shop)
- 3 tbsp sweet and spicy Asian sauce (Asian shop)
- 3 tsp Vegetable broth (instant)
- 2 tsp food starch
- 1 federal government chives
- 1 small lettuce
- 400 g Silken tofu

preparation

25 minutes

1. Mix the rice wine and soy sauce. Mix half of the mixture with the mince.
2. Peel and finely chop the ginger and garlic. Heat the oil in a wok or large saucepan. Fry the ginger and garlic in it, turning. Add Szechuan pepper and mince and stir-fry for about 5 minutes. Stir in the chili bean sauce, add 1 liter of water and the rest of the rice wine and soy sauce mixture. Stir in the broth, bring everything to the boil and simmer for about 5 minutes. Mix the starch with 1-2 tablespoons of cold water until smooth. Stir into the soup, bring to the boil and simmer for about 1 minute.
3. In the meantime, wash the chives, shake dry and cut into rolls. Clean the lettuce, wash it, drain it well and pluck it into pieces. Cut the tofu into cubes. Add the chives to the soup and warm for about 1 minute while stirring carefully. Divide the lettuce into four soup bowls. Pour the soup over the salad, serve.

Nutritional info

1 portion approx:

400 kcal27 g protein28 g fat6 g of carbohydrates

Thai salmon with radish salad

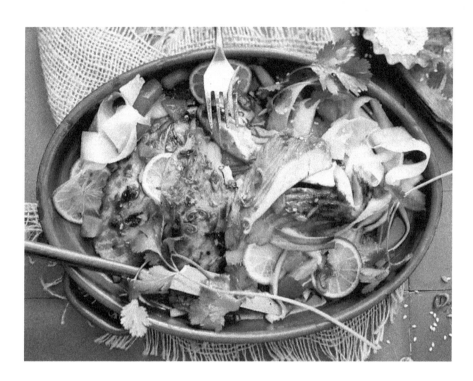

Ingredients For 4 people

- 1 piece (approx. 20 g each) ginger
- 2 Garlic cloves
- 2 red chili peppers
- 1 pole Lemongrass
- 6-8 tbsp Soy sauce
- Sugar, salt
- 1 federal government coriander
- 600 g Salmon fillet (skinless)
- 1 small radish
- 4th tomatoes
- 1 Organic lime
- 1 Red onion
- 4 tbsp oil

- 2 tbsp sesame
- Cling film, ice cubes

preparation

50 minutes (+ 45 minutes waiting time)

1. For the marinade, peel and finely chop the ginger and garlic. Clean the chilli, cut lengthways, core, wash and chop. Clean and wash lemongrass and cut into very fine rings. Bring lemongrass, ginger, garlic, half of the chilli, soy sauce and 1 teaspoon sugar to the boil and remove from the heat. Let cool down. Wash the coriander, shake dry and pluck the leaves. Chop the stalks and stir into the marinade.

2. Wash the salmon, pat dry and cut into 4 slices. Place the fish in a baking dish, pour the cooled sauce over it and sprinkle with half of the coriander leaves. Cover with cling film and refrigerate for about 1 hour.

3. In the meantime, peel the radish for the salad, wash it and cut lengthways into strips with a peeler. Chill the strips in approx. 1 liter of cold salted water (1 teaspoon of salt) with 1 handful of ice cubes for approx. 30 minutes.

4. Wash tomatoes and dice finely. Wash the lime in hot water, dry it and cut into thin slices. Peel the onion and cut into fine rings. Mix everything with the rest of the chilli and 2 tablespoons of oil.

5. Remove the salmon from the marinade and pat dry. Toast the sesame seeds in a large pan without fat for about 2 minutes, remove. Heat 2 tablespoons of oil in the pan and fry the salmon for 2-3 minutes on each side. Pour in the marinade and bring to the boil. Take the salmon off the stove. Drain the radish and mix with the tomato mix. Arrange the lettuce, salmon, sesame seeds and the rest of the coriander.

TIP: If you have toasted sesame oil in your cupboard, it should definitely be used for the tomatoes.

Nutritional info

1 portion approx:

480 kcal34 g protein33 g fat7 g of carbohydrates

Minty pea soup

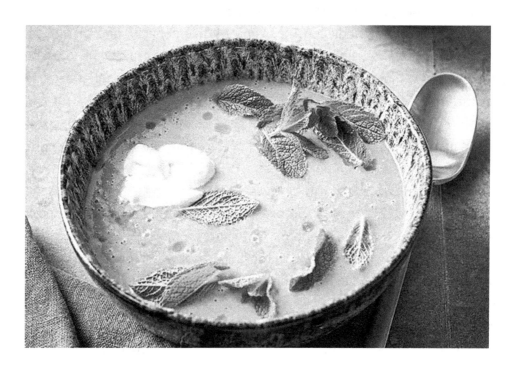

Ingredients For 4 people

- 1 onion
- 1 clove of garlic
- 2 tbsp olive oil
- 750 g Frozen peas
- 1 tbsp Vegetable broth (instant)
- 1 small bunch of mint
- 200 g Sour cream
- Salt pepper
- 1 tbsp Lime juice
- 1 / 2-1 tsp green tabasco

preparation

20 minutes

1. Peel and roughly dice the onion and garlic. Heat oil in a pot. Braise both in it. Add 1 liter of water and frozen peas, bring to the boil. Stir in the broth and simmer for about 5 minutes.
2. Wash the mint, shake dry, pull off the leaves. Add half to the soup and puree everything finely with a hand blender. Stir in half of the sour cream. Season to taste with salt, pepper, lime juice and Tabasco. Serve with the rest of the sour cream and mint.

Nutritional info

1 portion approx:

300 kcal11 g protein19 g fat19 g carbohydrates

Rice pan with savoy cabbage-paprika-vegetables and sour cream dip

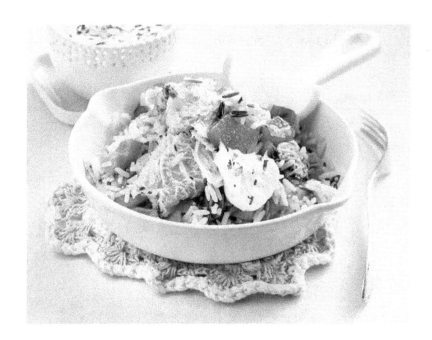

Ingredients For 1 people

- 1 untreated lemon
- 100 g Skimmed milk yogurt
- 1 tbsp frozen Italian herb mixture
- salt
- pepper
- sugar
- 50 g Wild rice mix
- 150 g Savoy cabbage
- 1/2 red pepper
- 1 tbsp olive oil

preparation

35 minutes

1 Wash the lemon with hot water, rub dry and tear off the zest of 1/4 lemon in zest. Halve the lemon, cut a quarter into 2 wedges. Use the rest otherwise. Squeeze out 1 column, stir in the yoghurt and lemon zest, except for something to sprinkle until smooth.

2 Add herbs, fold in, season with salt, pepper and sugar. Prepare wild rice mixture in boiling salted water according to the instructions on the packet. Clean and wash the savoy cabbage, cut out the hard core.

3 Cut the savoy cabbage leaves into pieces. Clean and wash the peppers and cut into pieces. Heat oil in a pan. Fry the savoy cabbage and paprika for 2-3 minutes, turning. Pour rice into a sieve, drain, add to vegetables and fry for about 2 minutes.

4 Season to taste with salt and pepper. Sprinkle the yogurt dip with the rest of the lemon zest. Add the remaining lemon wedge and dip.

Nutritional info

1 person approx:

350 kcal1470 kJ14 g protein11 g fat

Summer rolls with a sweet sesame dip

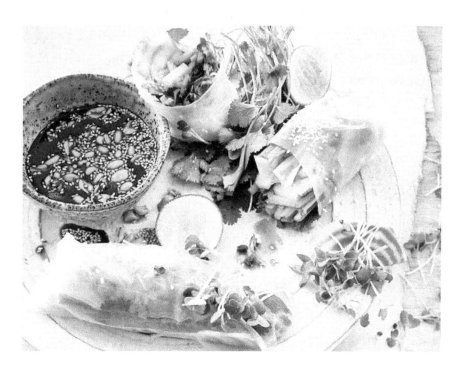

Ingredients For 4 people

- 1 Red onion
- 2 Carrots
- 1 Mini romaine lettuce
- 1/2 Cucumber
- 1 Ringlet beet (approx. 150 g; alternatively, beetroot)
- 1 federal government coriander
- 16 sheets (round) Rice paper (22 cm Ø)
- 50 g roasted peanuts
- 100 ml Soy sauce (e.g., ketjap manis)
- 1-2 tbsp Agave syrup
- 1 tbsp Rice vinegar
- 2 tsp sesame
- Organic lime
- 1 bed cress

preparation

45 minutes

1   Peel the onion and carrots and cut into fine strips. Clean the lettuce, wash, spin dry, cut into strips. Peel the cucumber and cut into strips. Peel and halve the beetroot and slice or cut into thin slices. Wash the coriander and shake dry.

2   Place rice paper sheets one after the other on a damp tea towel, brush evenly with approx. 5 tablespoons of water and soak for approx. 1 minute. Place some of the prepared ingredients in the middle of the rice paper. Sprinkle with a few peanuts each and roll up.

3   Mix the soy sauce, agave syrup and vinegar with 1 teaspoon sesame seeds and the rest of the peanuts. Wash lime in hot water, dry and cut into slices. Cut the cress from the bed. Arrange summer rolls, sauce and lime. Sprinkle with cress and the rest of the sesame seeds.

4   Place the filling in the middle as a wide strip on the soaked rice paper sheet. Fold the left and right rice paper edges over the filling. Lay the lower side on top. Now roll up tightly.

Nutritional info

1 portion approx:

400 kcal12 g protein15 g fat52 g of carbohydrates

Steak pan with honey balsamic vinegar

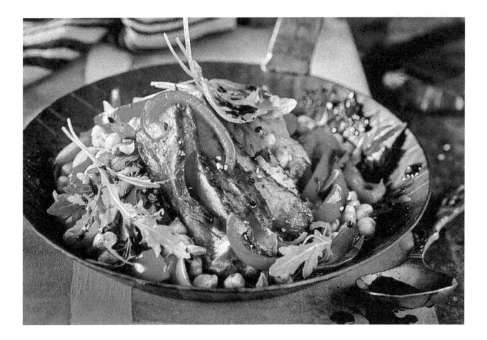

Ingredients For 2 people

- 360 g Rumpsteak
- 2 tbsp oil
- 1/2 can (s) (425 ml each) Chickpeas
- 1 red pepper
- 2 Red onions
- 2 tbsp Liquid honey
- 5 tbsp Balsamic vinegar
- Salt pepper
- 1 federal government arugula
- Aluminum foil

preparation

20 minutes

1. Pat the steak dry, rub 1 tablespoon of oil all around. Fry them vigorously on each side in a hot pan without fat for about 2 minutes.
2. Rinse the chickpeas with cold water and drain them. Clean and wash the peppers. Peel the onions. Cut the onions and peppers into thin strips.
3. Wrap the steak in foil and let it rest for about 5 minutes. Heat 1 tablespoon of oil in the pan. Fry the peppers, onions and chickpeas in it, turning. Stir in honey, deglaze with vinegar. Season with salt and pepper.
4. Clean and wash the rocket, shake dry and roughly pluck. Salt, pepper and slice the steak. Serve with rocket on the vegetable pan.

Nutritional info

1 portion approx:

400 kcal43 g protein15 g fat22 g of carbohydrates

Cauliflower Rice

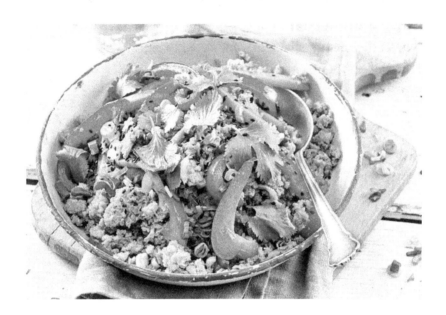

Ingredients For 4 people

- 800 g cauliflower
- 20 g fresh ginger
- red peppers
- Carrots
- 4th Spring onions
- stems coriander
- tbsp sesame oil
- tbsp Soy sauce
- Salt pepper
- 1 tsp Curry powder
- 4th Eggs (size M)
- 1 tbsp black sesame seeds

preparation

50 minutes

1. Clean the cauliflower, cut from the stalk in large florets and wash. Roughly grate the florets on a grater. Peel and finely dice the ginger. Wash and clean the peppers and cut into strips. Peel the carrots and cut into sticks. Wash and clean the spring onions and cut into fine rings. Wash the coriander, shake dry and pluck the leaves from the stems.
2. Heat 2 tablespoons of sesame oil in a large pan or wok. Fry the cauliflower rice in it for 3 -5 minutes while stirring. Add the ginger and deglaze with the soy sauce. Season with salt, pepper and curry powder. Heat 1 tablespoon of sesame oil in another pan, fry the paprika strips and carrot sticks for 3-5 minutes. Season with salt and pepper.
3. Whisk the eggs and pour over the cauliflower rice. Let the egg set while stirring. Add paprika, carrot and spring onion. Season to taste and serve in bowls. Garnish with coriander leaves and black sesame seeds and serve.

Nutritional info

1 portion approx:

280 kcal14 g protein16 g fat16 g of carbohydrates

CONCLUSION

Losing weight without exercise is possible and not necessarily more difficult than with physical activity. The basic requirement for sustainable weight loss is a healthy relationship with food. It shouldn't serve as a frustration killer or a pastime.

Above all else, rely on natural whole foods and avoid processed foods that have a higher calorie density than their volume suggests.

If you lack the willpower to say "no" to temptations in everyday life, develop strategies to avoid giving in. Prepare meals for yourself or deliberately make it more difficult to access sweets by not even putting them on your shopping list.

The ideal weight is not to be equated with a flawless dream figure. It's a medical value that tells you how much you should weigh based on your age, gender, and height. Give your body time to slowly settle down to a weight that is healthy and comfortable for you.

Find a way to eat a more balanced diet without viewing it as agony or compulsion. In the long run, you can actually lose weight without exercising.

CPSIA information can be obtained
at www.ICGtesting.com
Printed in the USA
BVHW010855250621
610445BV00003B/169